T0385321

THE GAME CHANGER

THE GAME CHANGER

Baroness Sue Campbell

with *Ben Dirs*

CONSTABLE

CONSTABLE

First published in Great Britain in 2025 by Constable

1 3 5 7 9 10 8 6 4 2

A CIP catalogue record for this book
is available from the British Library.

ISBN: 978-1-40872-085-1 (hardback)

Typeset in Bembo by Hewer Text UK Ltd, Edinburgh
Printed and bound in Great Britain by Clays Ltd, Elcograf S.p.A.

Papers used by Constable are from well-managed
forests and other responsible sources.

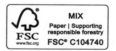

Constable
An imprint of
Little, Brown Book Group
Carmelite House
50 Victoria Embankment
London EC4Y 0DZ

The authorised representative
in the EEA is
Hachette Ireland
8 Castlecourt Centre, Dublin 15,
D15 XTP3, Ireland
(email: info@hbgi.ie)

An Hachette UK Company
www.hachette.co.uk

www.littlebrown.co.uk

For the many wonderful people along my journey who
have shaped my life for the better

Contents

Foreword

I don't think that there is anyone else in the last forty years who has made such a difference to British sport. Sue and I first met at Loughborough, where she had been appointed as the first full-time woman on the staff in the PE department and I was a student. We established a great friendship that has lasted over fifty years.

Sue was in the vanguard of delivering the performances that we witnessed in London and beyond in the Olympic and Paralympic Games in 2012. The London Games were a huge celebration for the entire country – and if we hadn't had those big unforgettable moments across so many different sports, I don't think people would still be talking about London as the best, most successful and most accessible Games of the modern era.

Earlier in her career, Sue headed up the National Coaching Foundation where she laid the foundation for the modernisation of coaching and the integration of sports science and medicine into coaching qualifications for all sports. Later her contribution to school sport as Chief Executive and then Chair of the Youth Sport Trust was world-beating. She established a national network of School Sport Partnerships that improved opportunities for every young person in schools across the country, transforming physical education and school sport. More recently she has had a seismic impact on women's football as Director of Women's Football at the Football Association, resulting in the biggest football success in my lifetime when the women's team won the European Championship in 2022.

Sue has been a role model, domestically and globally, as a female sports leader – a truly outstanding game changer.

Seb Coe, CH, KBE, 2024

Prologue

I can see Chloe Kelly now, hurtling towards me across the Wembley turf.

She leaps at me from about five feet away and I struggle to stay on my feet. Luckily, there now exists a wonderful picture of me and Chloe in a joyful embrace, rather than of both of us in an unsightly pile on the ground. The atmosphere in the stadium was electric, with 87,000 fans celebrating ecstatically – a noise I will not forget. My heart was racing with excitement as I realised that this was a landmark moment for the women's game in England.

A lot has happened in my life since Chloe scored the winning goal for England's Lionesses in the final of Euro 2022, but I can still feel that moment. I can also still touch it – because of what it meant to so many people.

That moment wasn't just about winning. It was also about human connection, the sharing of pure joy – a joy that is impossible to describe, a joy that will never fade. I'll be able to touch that moment for the rest of my days.

But that's not the only moment I can touch. I've so many of them, collected from a lifetime in sport: playing football with the boys when I should have been at school; playing backyard cricket with my dad until it was too dark to see the ball; the first time wearing a shirt bearing my country's name and flag; the pride of seeing teams I coached win (and win well); the pleasure of seeing the less privileged and the less inclined play sport at all; the exhilaration of seeing athletes I helped succeed on the world's biggest stages.

It hasn't all been milk and honey. I'll never forget being told I wasn't allowed to play football at school – bang went my dream of playing for England at Wembley. I still wince when I think about the time I made a presentation on my new plan for coach development to a roomful of the finest senior coaches in the country, all but one of them men, none of whom was convinced they needed what I was selling. It still pains me when I think of the destruction that was done to the school sports movement in this country, something that had taken many years to build. But those bad moments were just bumps in the road; nothing derailed my mission.

The mission? To change people's lives through sport, just as sport changed mine. Because while I ended up being a baroness, I wasn't exactly destined for the House of Lords from birth. In fact, if you'd told my mum and dad that I'd become a titled woman, they'd have thought you'd lost your mind.

At school I was a naughty little ginger-haired girl who was a massive underachiever. I had a passion for sport at a time when it was virtually impossible for women to make a living from it, unless you wanted to teach PE. But I was fortunate to have parents who understood that naughty little ginger girls who were not academic high-achievers could still succeed in life, which in turn fostered in me a moral purpose: to do everything in my power to make sure others could succeed, too.

In summary, I was a typical 'tomboy' who loved running, climbing, kicking and throwing – and other things most girls didn't do back then – and who grew into a woman with an unshakeable belief in the transformative power of sport.

You might think that someone with such a well-defined mission and strong moral purpose would travel through life as straight as an arrow speeding towards its target. In fact, I've been zigging and zagging for more than fifty years, between my passion for changing lives for the better through sport and my fascination with sporting excellence and helping talented people achieve their dreams.

You might also think that having had such a long career in sport – ranging from persuading inner-city unemployed young people to develop life skills through to helping Great Britain be more successful at the Olympics – I must have spread harmony wherever I've been. But that hasn't been the case at all.

Effective leadership often involves taking apart things that aren't working properly before putting them back together again so that they do. That means unsettling people who believe things are fine just as they are. It requires doing what you think is right, not what is popular or expedient. It takes optimism, perseverance, resilience, focus … And a lot of hard work.

I've been so engrossed in my mission for so long that I haven't had time for much else. But how many people have experienced what I've experienced through sport? And how many people can close their eyes and touch all the wonderful memories I can touch, as if they were happening here and now?

When I think of London 2012, I'm in the stadium on Super Saturday at the Olympics or Thriller Thursday at the Paralympics or wandering through the Olympic Park soaking up all that national pride. When I think of Euro 2022, I'm not just hugging Chloe, I can also feel the joy of more than 87,000 England fans inside Wembley Stadium. And I marvel at how lucky I've been.

It's a precious thing, my passion for sport. I hope it has made the world a bit better. And if a naughty little ginger-haired girl who underachieved at school can make the world better just by hard work, determination, caring and reaching out … then so can anyone.

1

Discovering your purpose

You need to remain open to discover your true purpose in
life that will be your 'north star' throughout your career

The bell sounds and the moment of truth has arrived – my first-ever lesson as a young twenty-one-year-old PE teacher. Class 4O, netball outside on a sunny day in early September. Surely a nice, easy introduction.

I arrive at the gym wearing my best tracksuit and shoes polished to within an inch of their lives. I've got a bag of netballs, bibs, and a comprehensive lesson plan attached to a clipboard. I'm ready for action. At least I think I am.

Five minutes go by and no one from 4O has appeared. I suddenly think, 'Oh no, have I misread the timetable? It's a split-site school – maybe I'm on the wrong site?', before belting towards the master timetable, worrying I'll be breaking the rules by running in the corridor (a cardinal sin in any school).

On my way there, I pass the toilets, which are a hive of activity. Loud chatter, laughing, singing. And then it hits me: 'Could that be 4O in there . . .?'

I open the toilet door, poke my head in and almost choke on the smoke. Through the haze, I can just about make out around twenty girls, all puffing away merrily.

Not one of them thinks to stub out their cigarette. They're completely unfazed. Unlike me. In three years at teacher training college, nobody ever told me what to do if you find your entire class in the toilet smoking cigarettes. Plus, all the girls are Black, a new experience for me.

I'm speechless in the face of such brazen defiance. Should I turn on my heel and leave them to it? Should I shout at them? Eventually I ask, 'Are you 4O?' And one of them replies, 'Yeah. Who are you?'

'I'm your PE teacher.'

'We don't do PE, Miss.'

'Pardon?'

'We don't do PE. Breaks your nails.'

I have deduced that shouting at them isn't going to make any difference – not that I have the energy to shout anyway. I feel flummoxed and feeble, and suddenly find myself sitting on the floor. It's not a premeditated ploy – 'to get down with the girls' – but I am honestly feeling light-headed.

One of them says, 'Miss, you look rough, do you want a cigarette?' I politely tell her no, while thinking, 'What am I doing? If a member of staff walks in now, my teaching career is done, before I've taught a single lesson.'

Then something unexpected happens – they all sit down on the floor with me. And we start to talk. Whatever question I ask, they're only too happy to answer me, with a lot of swearing thrown in. Maybe I should tell them to mind their language, but I don't think it will be too helpful in this situation. Better to let them talk freely, if that means getting to know them better.

Having expanded on their reasons for not doing PE – broken nails, messed-up hair, sweat, unflattering kit – I ask them what they do like to do when they're not at school. At first, I wish I hadn't asked, because they tell me things I don't really want to hear. I thought I was worldly, but I'm nothing like these girls. They may only be fourteen, but they're living very adult lives.

'What do you have most fun doing?' I ask.

'Clubbing,' comes the reply.

'So you like to dance?' I say.

With that, a couple of the girls get up off the floor and start demonstrating their moves. I love to dance, too, so decide to join in. Soon, the toilet is an impromptu disco, with everyone on their feet, singing and swaying.

'So,' I say, 'how about we dance next week, instead of playing netball?'

'Are you serious, Miss?'

'Yes. Tell you what, I'll bring a record player and you bring some music.'

'Do we have to change, Miss?'

'No. As long as you understand that you can't smoke and you'll have to take off your shoes, so you don't scuff the new parquet floor in the gym.'

The following week, I turn up with a record player instead of balls and bibs. The girls don't show up on time, but they do turn up eventually, with a range of music. And while they dance, I sit on a pile of mats in the corner, writing lesson plans. Is this what I'm being paid to do? No. Should I be doing something more constructive? Probably. But at least they're in the gym, enjoying themselves while exercising, instead of smoking in the toilet.

After a while, one of the girls comes over and says, 'Miss, we're a bit bored.'

'Want to play netball?' I reply.

'No, Miss! We want to form a dance group!'

'Erm ... OK, but you're going to have to lead it, because this music isn't really my thing, and I'm not much of a dancer anyway.'

I meet with the girl during lunch breaks to plan sessions, and it soon becomes clear that she can't read very well. So we start reading together, discussing what each word means, and she improves bit by bit. She's a pleasure to work with – all that attitude from our first encounter in the toilet has melted away.

Many of the qualities you need to be the leader of a gang – which was essentially what this girl was – are the same you need to be an effective leader of people on a more positive mission. You need charisma, standards, passion and a good work ethic, and this girl has all those qualities in spades. As a result, her classmates listen to her, like they never listen to me. I tell her that she's a better teacher than me, and I mean it.

With my support, she knocks her classmates into shape. And over the coming weeks and months, the girls of 4O change before my eyes. They don't just become better dancers who win accolades, they start to feel good about themselves. For maybe the first time, they have a sense of pride. And it suddenly hits me: the best people to lead young people are young people. Find a youngster with the right attitude and the others will follow.

Without a doubt, it's the awakening of my mission. Before meeting those girls, I thought my job was to teach netball, hockey, tennis and athletics. But I begin to understand that education is not just about learning, it's about empowerment and facilitation, enabling young people to gain the confidence and self-esteem to bring out the best in themselves. This experience was like a new dawning – a realisation that I had in my hands the power to change lives through and in sport. I have had many roles since that day, but I have only had one mission.

You cannot force a child to learn, so it's a teacher's job to create an environment in which they *want* to learn. And that environment might not be one the teacher is familiar with – like dancing instead of netball – but great teachers teach young people more than just the subject matter laid out in the curriculum.

I realise I have a higher purpose: that if I listen carefully and work collaboratively, I can actually change young lives through physical activity. It's an awakening: in every child is a magic spark – it's my job to find it.

2

Be history – or make history

*When we do not succeed, we have a choice either
to give up or to find the resolve to go again*

Despite our very different backgrounds, I felt I knew those
girls from class 4O. It's not as if I had some special insight,
rather that there was something about their defiance I
recognised.

Mum and Dad both came from humble backgrounds and
left school early, with no qualifications whatsoever. But what
they lacked in book-smarts they more than made up for in
people skills.

Mum started out as a hairdresser. When she was learning
her trade, her weekly bus fare from her home in Long Eaton
to Nottingham was three shillings, and she only earned two
shillings and sixpence. Her dad would give her a tanner, as
we used to call a sixpence, to make up for the loss.

After a while, her boss Mr Smith suggested she start up on
her own, so she opened a place in Long Eaton. She was

obviously an excellent hairdresser, very popular, as well as entrepreneurial, and before long she also had salons in Beeston and Ilkeston. This was quite unusual for a woman in the 1940s. Later, as I made my own way in the professional world, I realised what a remarkable achievement it was to have the courage and determination to succeed as a woman in business.

Dad started off working as a delivery boy for the local Co-op before becoming a manager. And when Mum had me, five years after my sister Gill, Dad took over the running of the salons and Mum concentrated on hairdressing. They were both charming and able to communicate with anybody. Walking with Dad across the green in Long Eaton, from the shop to the Spot Café, seemed to take forever because of all the people wanting to talk to him.

Probably because they'd had so little education themselves, Mum and Dad put a lot of emphasis on ours. So despite living in Chilwell, Gill and I were sent off to Dorothy Grant's, a private girls' school in nearby Beeston. We had to wear straw boaters, which wasn't really me. And while Gill was very well behaved and academic, school life was a bit more complicated for me.

My class teacher was a wonderful woman called Mrs Jury. She introduced me to netball, except I don't think she'd read the rulebook, so we could tackle people. Looking back, it was more like rugby.

I don't remember ever sitting in a classroom with Mrs Jury – we seemed to learn everything by moving and doing, usually outdoors. But I was a ginger-haired, freckled tomboy, whose best friends were boys. As much as I loved full-contact netball, I spent a lot of time staring out of the classroom window wishing I was doing something else, something active, maybe climbing trees, or anything involving a ball.

After school, I'd play cricket with Dad, much to Mrs North's fury, because I'd constantly be hitting the ball into her garden next door. Dad would say to me, 'You'd better knock on her door, you've got a better chance of getting it back than me.'

Dad painted targets on the garage door for my football practice – three at the top, three at the bottom – and he'd say to me, 'You've got to hit those spots fifty times before you come in for your tea.' Sometimes, I'd come in and he'd say, 'Have you cheated?' 'Maybe I didn't quite get fifty . . .' 'It's all right, you can have your tea anyway – but keep working on it . . .'

Dad was originally from Manchester, which is why I've supported Manchester United all my life. When I was too small to know better, he convinced me that United had moved to Nottingham, so that whenever we watched Nottingham Forest at the City Ground, I thought I was watching the famous 'Busby Babes' . . . until I worked out the final scores didn't match!

Dad and I had some epic kickabouts in our back garden, and if he was busy with work, and my friends Brian Carrier and Geoffrey Stafford weren't allowed out to play, I'd kick a ball against a wall for hours on my own, blissfully happy.

Our house was at the top of Farm Road, which was a long, winding, downhill road that connected with Hall Drive. Brian and I would roller-skate that circuit regularly, and we could get round it fast. We'd race each other hell for leather on opposite pavements and often return home with bloody knees and grazed elbows. How we didn't kill ourselves I do not know.

My boy mates all went to the local Chilwell primary school, and when I said to Brian one day, 'I don't get to play much football nowadays,' he replied, 'Oh, we play all the time. Before school, break time, lunch time, after school.' I thought for a moment, before saying, 'That's why you're getting much better than me. I need to do what you're doing.'

The following week, I started getting off the bus early and going to their school instead of mine, playing football and hiding in bushes while they were in classes. Eventually, someone from Dorothy Grant's rang my parents to ask where I'd been. Mum and Dad were baffled, as they'd been putting me on the bus every morning. So the next day Dad followed me and all was revealed. When he sat me down and asked what was going on, I told him I wanted to play football with all my friends. And instead of being angry, like a lot of dads would, he took me out of Dorothy Grant's and enrolled me in Chilwell primary school.

I've always been a storyteller, and I know exactly where I got that from. After playing football with Brian and Geoffrey, they'd often say to me, 'Is your dad home? It would be good to come round and hear one of his stories.' And Dad would sit us round the table and treat us to a few of his greatest yarns.

His stories were a mix of real happenings and elaboration – full of life, wise and often funny – because if they'd been delivered like a lecture or sermon, we wouldn't have listened. They always had a great punchline, but without the build-up, we'd probably have missed the point, which is something I've never forgotten. Whenever I present to an audience, I'm all about storytelling, because that's how you get people to engage with your message.

Mum and Dad weren't just keen on us getting a classroom education, they also wanted us to experience the world far beyond Nottinghamshire.

Dad believed the seaside air was especially good for you (something to do with the ozone), so he'd take us to the coast at Skegness once a month, even in the middle of winter. Sometimes we'd turn up and be just about the only people there, but we'd spend all day on the beach regardless, even if it was freezing cold and blowing a hooley.

We also played golf on the putting green – Dad played off scratch and Mum wasn't bad either. Dad would say, 'Mum and I will have to keep missing until you get one in, because if we beat you, the rest of the day will be miserable.' I was a typical redhead, very competitive and a bad loser when it came to sport.

We'd travel further afield every summer, often down to Newquay in Cornwall, but sometimes over to France,

Switzerland or even Italy, the kinds of holidays most people didn't go on in those days, especially families from Chilwell.

In Newquay, they'd let me stay up late and go to dances, where I'd stand on Dad's feet and he'd waltz me around the floor. In Interlaken, we caught a train to the top of the mountain and hired skis. I fell on the way down, couldn't get back up and threw my skis to the ground in a fit of pique. We water-skied in Neuchâtel. In Rouen, we saw where Joan of Arc was burnt at the stake.

They're all precious memories, even the minor disasters. Like the time Mum and Dad went for a walk in Paris, got hopelessly lost and forgot what hotel we were staying in. Gill and I worried that they'd fallen into the Seine. Or the holiday that began with Mum backing the car into the gate and knocking down the wall at the front of the house. When Dad finally turned up, having been delayed in the shop, he took one look at the wall and said, 'We're not mending that now,' before jumping in the car and stepping on the gas.

Mum and Dad wanted to show us what was possible and for us to have a go at everything. In doing so, they encouraged me to become someone who wasn't afraid of pushing the boundaries and going to new places, both literally and metaphorically.

I somehow passed my 11-plus exam and made it to Long Eaton Grammar School, where I was put in class 1D, for pupils who had scraped through the exam.

Thankfully, Dad's sister, Auntie Kitty, was very clever. Having stayed on at school and attended the prestigious Manchester Grammar School, she decided to become a secretary rather than a teacher, which were just about the only two options for an educated woman in that era. She worked for the chief education officer at Nottinghamshire County Council, but also found time to support me to do my homework. She lived next door to us, so I'd go round and say, 'I've got this thing to do and I don't really understand it,' and she'd always reply, 'Go on then, let's sort it together . . .'

Unlike me, my sister Gill was studious, and very good at maths and science. After doing her A-levels, she went off to university to study mathematics in London, but only stayed a term. You have to be pretty headstrong to work hard enough to get into university and then decide it's not for you after all, especially as a young woman back then, but Mum and Dad supported her decision.

Next thing we knew, Gill applied to be an air traffic controller (she'd been obsessed with Airfix planes as a child – I remember Mum taking them down from her bedroom ceiling and washing them in the bath – Gill was not amused and had to glue them back together again). At her interview, Gill was told that they only accepted men, and she replied, 'Why?' They didn't have a good reason, so Gill became one of the first female air traffic controllers in the country.

Like Gill, I was wilful. Unlike Gill, I was a noisy, disruptive child with no interest in books. I spent most of my time in class staring longingly at the playing fields or sitting at the back and being a constant nuisance. I drove many of my teachers to distraction but they kept persevering with me! Outstanding teachers keep working with every pupil whatever challenges they present. Teachers were always asking, 'Why aren't you more like your sister?' I'd think, 'Because I'm not my sister.' I was bored in class. I didn't like sitting still – and still don't. I wanted, and want, to be moving all the time.

If I was in trouble, which was often, I'd head straight to our Long Eaton shop after school and knock on the window. When Dad appeared, he'd put his arm around me and we'd walk across the green to the Spot Café, where he'd listen to all my problems and put them into perspective over a pot of tea.

One day, I knocked on the window and told Dad I'd got my school report. Usually, Mum would read my report to Dad, because his reading wasn't the best, and he'd sign it. But on this occasion my report was so bad I didn't dare take it home.

Dad must have known something was wrong, but he played along and asked me to read it to him, 'like your mum normally does'. And off we went to the Spot Café, where I proceeded to make it all up. I told him I got an A in maths, which the teacher thought was an outstanding effort; that I got a B in English, but was trying hard; that I also got a B in German, which the long-suffering Mr Aldridge was thrilled about. In fact, I'd got Cs, Ds and Es all the way down, except for PE, which I'd actually got an A in and didn't have to lie about.

When I'd finished, Dad picked up his pen and looked like he was going to sign. But then he looked at me and said, 'This is your father signing this. Do you know what this means? Do you really want me to?' I went red and my eyes started to fill with tears. Then Dad said, 'Do you want to tell me what it really says?'

Between heaving sobs, I read Dad the horrible truth. By the end, my cheeks were wet with tears. I was looking for sympathy, of course. Then I said, 'Are you really cross with me?' and Dad replied, 'Only because you fibbed.'

I told him how hopeless I was, that I was never going to amount to anything, and he looked me straight in the eye and said, 'Sue Campbell, you will be whatever you want to be. You just haven't decided what it is yet.'

What brilliant timing. Whereas many dads would have told their daughters to stop messing about and knuckle down, or melted in the face of their tears, my dad delved deeper and quickly realised that my terrible report wasn't a complete picture of who I was, just a snapshot of what I'd done over a short period of time. So instead of getting angry or upset, Dad chose to empower me. He was essentially saying, 'You have to find your own path and follow it.'

What I really wanted to be was a footballer, but girls didn't play football at the grammar school. My heart sank when they told me that, because I honestly thought I was going to play for England. And even if you did have sporting talent, playing sport for a living was a pipe dream for most women in the 1960s, and would remain so for the next half a century.

But a lack of career opportunities in sport did nothing to dampen my enthusiasm. I was in both the netball and hockey teams and excelled at athletics. Ron and Sheila Bassett, husband-and-wife PE teachers at the grammar school, were really passionate about their subject and demanded high standards. They also realised that I had something a bit different. I became almost part of their family and even used to walk their dog, who I adored.

One day, when I was fourteen and languishing in class 3C, Sheila asked me what I was going to do with my life. 'I haven't decided yet,' I said. 'Play sport?'

Sheila replied, 'You're not going to earn a living doing that, however good you are. But you could become a PE teacher like me.'

'Sounds great. What do I have to do to be a PE teacher?'

'Well, for starters, you need to start sitting at the front of class and doing some learning.'

That little chat with Sheila was the springboard for the rest of my life. I never became academic, but I became a more thoughtful student, got stuck into schoolwork and revised for exams. And from 3C, I graduated to 4B.

Sheila started using me to assist with lessons – 'I'll take this group, Sue, you take that group over there' – and I loved the feeling of helping others, honing their ability and getting them to play better. I also started playing hockey with her for Ripley Ladies. I'd turn out for the school team on

Saturday mornings, dash home for Mum's stew and chips, before Sheila would pick me up and whisk me off to somewhere or other in the Midlands. I'd be absolutely done in by the end of the second game, but I loved it.

Dad would watch me play, and while he'd never swung a hockey stick in anger, he wasn't averse to giving his two penn'orth on the game. At the time, hockey tactics were very standardised. A team would always have five forwards, three halves, two backs and a goalie, and the two wings would stay in the tramlines, to give the team width, like in football. After one game, which we won, I was naturally quite excited. But Dad said to me, 'Well done, that was really good. But can I ask you something? What were you doing?'

'I was playing left wing.'

'But you never got the ball. You were just running up and down the side.'

'Yes, because I'm left wing.'

'But surely you need to get the ball now and again?'

He wasn't criticising me: he genuinely wanted to understand why we were playing how we were. And to be fair, he was years ahead of his time, because hockey, like football, has since evolved into a far more fluid game.

It was while playing for Midlands Hockey that I first met the irrepressible Rachel Heyhoe. Rachel was on her way to becoming one of the few female household names in British sport, but as a cricketer rather than a hockey player (although she did play as a goalkeeper for England).

I'd never known anybody tell stories like Rachel, although many of them weren't really for a teenage girl's ears (ironically, she taught PE at a grammar school in Wolverhampton). Her humour was right on the edge, to say the least. I remember listening to her and thinking, 'Wow, this woman is amazing . . .'

Rachel was a dynamo and a trailblazer, years ahead of her time. She didn't care who she offended and was relentless in the pursuit of getting what she wanted, be that scoring runs, getting women's cricket in the news, or simply earning the respect of the English cricket establishment (her original application for membership of the MCC was rejected, because the club was then male-only, but she was one of the first ten women to be admitted in 1999).

Having followed Rachel's long and wildly successful cricket career, the tables were turned when, in 2011, she followed me into the House of Lords as Baroness Heyhoe Flint. She still had the same energy as when we first met in the 1960s, although, mercifully, her stories weren't quite as risqué.

In my final two years at secondary school my weekends were just full of sport. After playing hockey all day on Saturday, on Sunday morning Dad would take me to train at Derby Ladies Athletics Club in Spondon. He would drop me off, head to the garden centre, and pick me up when I was done. And with the support of my coach, I made great strides as an athlete. He even taught me how to use weights in the gym, which was unusual for girls in the 1960s, when muscly women weren't in vogue.

I did the pentathlon, which was the precursor to the heptathlon (80m hurdles, long jump, shot put, high jump, 200m). I was a good all-rounder but not brilliant at any of the events, and I had a habit of dismantling the hurdles. My coach would say to me, 'Drive at the hurdle!', and I'd forget that you were supposed to go over it rather than straight through it. I even trained alongside David Hemery and his amazing coach at Crystal Palace a few times. David remains a good friend to this day.

I was also a pretty good discus thrower, I had a natural throwing arm and could get a good distance with discus, javelin and shot. I'd practise in the cattle field opposite our house, and Dad (my personal coach) would bring a bucket of water along, so he could wash the discus off whenever it landed in a cowpat.

The problem with discus is, if you get nervous and your arm locks at the wrong time, it tends to land outside the sector, which means it's a no-throw. And I was so nervous the first two years I competed for Derbyshire schools in the English Schools' Athletics Championships that I recorded three no-throws on both occasions.

Dad was watching through the window when I returned home after the second event, and saw me lift the lid off the dustbin, throw my kitbag in and slam the lid back down. He said to Mum, 'I think you better leave this to me.'

When I walked in the kitchen, Dad was sitting at the table, with Mum nowhere to be seen.

'No good?' he said.

'No,' I replied. 'Three bloomin' no-throws again.'

'I've seen you throw your kitbag in the bin. Is that it, then? You're done?'

'Yep. I'm done, I did all that training and achieved nothing.'

'In years to come, you'll look back and feel bad about the fact you gave up.'

'I'm not giving up!'

'Looks that way to me.'

There wasn't much I could say to that, because he was right. Then, after one of his wise pauses, he said, 'Sue, your mum and I will love you whatever you choose to do. But in life, you can either be history or you can make history. That's your choice.'

He would have been a brilliant sports psychologist. He certainly knew how to keep me on the straight and narrow, and I wasn't an easy young woman to handle.

I went straight outside and fished my kitbag from the bin. It stank, but my retirement was at an end. The following year, I won the English Schools' discus title with my very first throw. Whack! Straight down the middle.

Although I never blossomed into much of a scholar the headmaster Mr Gray must have seen something in me, because he made me head girl. At the time, I didn't understand why, because head girls and boys tended to be academic high-achievers, and I was far too busy doing other things. Then again, I was captain of netball and hockey, so must have displayed resilience, determination and leadership.

I failed all my A-levels, but thankfully you only needed five O-levels to get into Bedford College of Physical Education, because in those days they weren't considered degree courses. Nowadays, you wouldn't get anywhere near a teacher training college without A-levels. And, looking back, there must have been times when Bedford wondered why they hadn't set their standards higher . . .

3

Valuing everyone

*Every individual needs to feel a sense of
belonging and feel appreciated*

I was at Bedford to learn how to teach PE, but we also played an awful lot of sport. I'd get up at the crack of dawn, go to swimming class, shower, grab a drink, cycle to the hockey pitch, play a match, cycle back to campus, grab some lunch, go to gymnastics class, grab a drink, cycle to the netball court, play a match, cycle back to campus, grab dinner . . . And repeat. It was bliss.

However, I wouldn't want you to think that Bedford was a glorified holiday camp, because it was far from that. I believe Bedford helped lay the foundations for the professional skills that have served me well throughout my working life.

The principal was an amazing Yorkshire woman called Eileen Alexander, who trained PT instructors during the Second World War before taking charge at Bedford in 1951.

Eileen had a reputation as a fearsome character, and in some respects ran Bedford with a rod of iron (you'd hear her imploring students to stop slouching, stand taller and achieve excellence in everything they did). But she'd created an incredibly professional environment, and she drilled into us the maxim 'Prepare well, deliver, review'. Anywhere I've ever worked, colleagues have rolled their eyes when I've repeated that – 'Oh no, not that again . . .' Cut me in half and it would be written right through me like a stick of rock.

At school, I struggled to learn through traditional methods, which almost always involved a teacher explaining things with a blackboard and a stick of chalk. And if they'd tried to teach me about anatomy and kinesiology (the scientific study of human body movement), I'd have struggled. But at Bedford, I was ready to learn and understand how the body worked and how I could train my body to achieve my potential. I began to understand that training needed to be specific to meet the challenges of the sport I was doing if it was to have the desired effect. I began analysing my sport more carefully and designing purpose-built programmes to ensure that I had the endurance, strength and flexibility alongside my technical and tactical skills to play at my very best.

Young people learn in many different ways, and I learned best through applied practice. So understanding how to perform any skill requires having an in-depth knowledge of the muscles involved and how to train to increase the strength and elasticity of those muscles to help you improve your performance. If a teacher had mentioned anatomy or kinesiology in a classroom at school, I'd immediately have switched off. But at Bedford, there was a direct link between the subjects and what I loved doing, which made it engaging. When the student is ready the teacher appears!

The more I understood about how my body worked, the better I got at training myself. Every night, I'd go to the gym with a friend, Pam Milner, having probably already done sessions in swimming and gymnastics, and played hockey or netball. We'd set up a circuit, including weights or parallel bars to build up our strength and stamina, put some Stevie Wonder on the stereo, and away we'd go. Last Christmas, Pam sent me a message: 'I'll never forget those sessions in the gym at Bedford, "For Once in My Life" blasting out.'

Because we were all like-minded people who loved physical activity – gymnasts, swimmers, netball players, dancers – and generally being busy, we also had an enormous amount of fun in our free time. Everyone was competitive, wanted to get in the team and be the best, but we were a tribe. We recently met up in London, as we try to do every year, and we all went back to our teenage years, despite all now being in our seventies. Much of the chat centred on the awful things we got up to at Bedford, whether it was filling the local fountain with washing powder, or the time we went for a midnight swim, not knowing that the pool had been drained. Thank goodness nobody dived in, although someone did jump in and sprain both ankles. We were meant to be home before curfew and I got caught trying to shove the injured party through a window.

I wasn't a great gymnast or dancer, but I was good at athletics and games. I built a wide group of friends and became popular with my fellow students, so at the end of my second year, they voted to make me senior student. Just as at school, people were seeing things in me – although the exacting Eileen Alexander wasn't sold on the idea at first.

It was a college tradition that once appointed, the senior student, wearing the famous Bedford cape, would walk to the principal's office and knock three times, a bit like Black Rod at the State Opening of Parliament. All very formal. On entering, I informed Eileen that I was her new senior student, and she looked at me over her half-moon glasses and said, 'My oh my, this is going to be an interesting year . . .'

One of the first things I did as senior student was try to persuade Eileen to open a bar in the student union. Her initial response was, 'Sue, dear, everyone will get drunk!' 'No, no, no,' I replied, 'we'll run the bar and keep on top of things . . .' I'm sure some drunkenness went on, but Eileen would sometimes come down and have a gin and tonic with us. Over the year she and I had many discussions and disagreements, but my respect for her and all she stood for grew and grew. Eileen saw me as a positive disrupter driving change on behalf of my fellow students. We established a friendship that would last a lifetime until her death, aged 102, in 2014.

During my time at Bedford, I captained the England Under-21s netball team, became British universities pentathlon champion (track and field version), and began to take a range of coaching qualifications in a number of sports.

Meanwhile, Eileen had convinced Cambridge University to take nine Bedford students for a pilot Bachelor of Education degree, and I was on the list (until then, Bedford students had graduated with a teaching certificate, which Eileen believed was unfair given the amount of study involved).

What I didn't know was that, despite being senior student, I was only ninth on the list (yes, I was good at sport, and showed promise as a teacher, but I still wasn't very strong academically). So when Cambridge decided that they were only going to take seven students from Bedford, I was informed I was not going.

That was a blow, for a couple of reasons. First, a Cambridge degree would have been a wonderful learning experience and a recognition for me and others of the three-year extensive programme we had undertaken at Bedford. Second, it was a last-minute decision, so I hadn't applied for teaching jobs, and what was left was extremely limited.

But as it turned out, fate had dealt me a great hand.

A ladies' college offered me a job, which would have involved teaching lacrosse. Not for me – I could barely play the game myself. But I was also offered a job at Whalley Range High School, on the outskirts of Manchester city centre, close to where Dad was born. Life turns corners you didn't even know were there, and being offered and accepting that job was probably one of the most important things that ever happened to me.

Once upon a time, Whalley Range was a well-to-do suburb, an escape from the deprivation and congestion of

Manchester's industrial centre. But after the Second World War, the area fell into decline. Wealthier families moved further afield, once-grand houses fell into disrepair and Whalley Range became known for its bedsits and red-light district.

I moved into a bedsit a few hundred yards from the red-light district. A man who made good omelettes lived downstairs, beneath the launderette, but that was about the only thing to recommend it. It had a bed, a small table and a sink, and when Mum came to visit, she took one look at the place and was very shocked. She went out and bought a bottle of Dettol and various other cleaning products, but even after scrubbing and polishing for hours, she said to me, 'Surely you can do better than this?' 'No, Mum,' I replied, 'I really can't.' If I remember rightly, my first salary was about £18 a week, or £900 a year.

Before moving to Whalley Range, I'd seen almost nothing of the massive deprivation faced by some families and young people in British society. I suddenly realised that there were people who had a daily battle to survive, to feed their families and to provide the love and support necessary to raise their children. The deprivation was genuinely shocking, and I was scared walking the streets, particularly at night. It was a deeply uncomfortable situation, and for the first few months I often wondered how I was going to cope.

In 1967, a few years before I joined, Whalley Range Grammar School became the comprehensive Whalley

Range High School, which meant incorporating Moss Side Secondary School, which was very rundown.

The deprivation in Moss Side was on a whole different level. The area had been badly bombed during the war, and the council began so-called slum clearances in the 1960s, demolishing most of the terraced houses that the Luftwaffe had missed and replacing them with council houses and flats. It was a good idea on paper, but it tore the heart out of the community. By the 1980s, Moss Side was mostly known for gangs, drugs and shootings.

Nobody at Whalley Range Grammar School had been ready for the transition, and a rather crude compromise was hatched. In her wisdom, the head teacher decided to bring the older secondary-school pupils into the former grammar school, to be taught by the grammar-school teachers, and match the secondary-school teachers with the younger pupils at the old secondary school.

Many of the grammar-school teachers had no experience of dealing with pupils who were less academic and not engaged in learning in the traditional way. They weren't bad teachers, but they struggled to adapt to a very different learning environment.

They had spent many years teaching science, French and Latin, Dickens and Shakespeare, to pupils who wanted to learn. Now, they were trying to teach those subjects to pupils who were unable to manage the basics of reading and writing, and who challenged their authority. I remember one teacher telling me about a field trip which had spiralled out of control. One of the teachers had called one of the pupils a name, and that evening they had all come down for dinner stark naked, in solidarity. It was a tough environment to suddenly find yourself in as a teacher. No wonder some of them were struggling to cope.

For my part, I had never encountered young women with so many challenges and who found their meaning in all the wrong places. When I was at Bedford, I taught at the Dame Alice Harpur School, where all the pupils dressed, spoke and behaved impeccably. In contrast, some of the girls at Whalley Range High School had very grown-up lifestyles. A few of them were already earning a living in the red-light district. Life was so difficult for many of them that education wasn't even on their radar, let alone Dickens and Shakespeare.

There were girls at Whalley Range High School who wanted to learn. So while I never did get class 4O to play netball, we did have some good teams, largely made up of girls from more middle-class backgrounds. But class 4O was full of girls for whom the model of education and leadership at the school just didn't work. Over time, they'd become more and more rebellious, while their teachers had become more inclined to let them do whatever they wanted, including smoke in the toilets when they should have been in lessons.

To be fair, if I had been teaching for ten years, I would not have sat on the floor of that toilet and started chatting. Like most of the other teachers, I would probably have yelled at them and left it at that. Thank goodness I was what I was, an inexperienced teacher in the dark, trying to grope my way towards solutions. I don't know if those girls saw me as a soft touch, but they did sense that I wanted to negotiate a solution, not impose one. And they went from being sullen and defensive, almost gang-like in their demeanour, to opening up about all sorts of things.

One thing I'd always been good at was asking questions, and I asked a lot of them. And it soon became clear that it wasn't just PE they didn't like: they hated everything about the place. They felt that Whalley Range, with its traditional, grammar-school curriculum, wasn't for them. And they seemed very aware that the old grammar-school teachers, few of whom asked questions about their lives, didn't want them to be there either.

Up to that point, sport had just been an incredible way to express who I was in the world. I simply thought that physical activity was thrilling and healthy, and I wanted the children I taught to have fun and be healthy too. I'd never thought of sport as a potential vehicle to change lives for the better.

One day, the head teacher told me to take a particularly naughty girl home. When we got in my car, she pleaded with me not to. I told her everything was going to be OK and that I'd smooth things over with her mum. I thought the girl was worried that her mum would be cross and give her a telling off, but her mum was actually a lady of the night and had a visitor, so she was terrified I'd see what was going on and somehow judge her.

I discovered that she was the eldest child, with three younger siblings, and the reason she kept getting detentions for being late and sneaking out early was because she had to dress the younger children every morning, drop them off at school, collect them afterwards and take them home. Meanwhile, her mum was doing what she felt she needed to do to put food on the table and keep a roof over their heads.

Nowadays, some schools have counsellors who have the time to get to know each child and understand their particular circumstances, but none of her teachers had time to delve into her problems. She didn't behave herself and meet the school's standards, so she got punished.

In an attempt to give this girl her own outlet I started taking her to Stretford Athletics Club, where I trained every Tuesday and Thursday (in those days, you could put a pupil in your car and take them places, no questions asked). And it turned out that she was a good athlete. I don't know what happened to her after she left school, but at least I know she made some good friends and perhaps it gave her some hope of a different future.

As for the girl who converted class 4O into a dance group, she didn't end up teaching dance for a living. But after leaving school with no qualifications, she studied at college and went on to work for the NHS. If you think the worst of a child, you'll probably get the worst. But I like to think that by listening to that girl, I had a positive effect on her, and made her realise that she could turn her flair for leadership into something positive.

I'm reminded of the film *Kes*, about a Yorkshire lad called Billy Casper who is bullied at home, has no interest in school and seems a lost cause. When Billy learns falconry, it gives his life meaning and broadens his horizons. In one scene, Billy's English teacher persuades him to give a talk about falconry in class, and it's the first time Billy has ever felt heard and been praised.

Kes is about the folly of a 'one size fits all' education system that doesn't cater for children who aren't academic but might have other useful skills. It's about the terrible waste of so many people and so much potential. And it's a tantalising glimpse of what can happen if just one curious adult identifies and validates just one child's passion and encourages him or her to run with it.

I'll be forever grateful to Whalley Range High School and the girls I met there. I often say that I learned more from them than they learned from me. They made me realise that my job as a teacher was to identify potential and invest in it; to provide children with an opportunity to feel good about themselves, valued, seen and heard. And they showed me that to achieve anything in life, you've got to ask questions, listen to people and at least try to understand.

4

Your greatest strength can be your greatest weakness

Know yourself well because what drives
you can also bring you down

Not long after I started teaching in Manchester when I was twenty-one, Dad became ill. First he had jaundice, then they discovered he had lung cancer. Like many men back then, even the sporty ones, he'd been smoking since he was a boy.

I'd drive home at weekends, across the Peak District and down the M1 through Derbyshire. And as time went on, it became obvious that there wasn't going to be a happy outcome.

Dad had a terrible fear of going into hospital, so we converted the lounge, where Mum nursed him. Towards the end, Dad was so heavily dosed up on various medications that he was hardly ever awake. Then, a couple of years after being diagnosed, he passed away. The wise, kind, gregarious man who had allowed me to be the person I wanted to be and laid the foundations on which I was beginning to build my life's work, was gone. The challenge was that I was so focused on Mum at first that I did not allow myself time to grieve. It was only later that I began to deal with this enormous loss. Maybe by burying it I made it worse – we will never know. But I do know that grief has to be confronted or it has the potential to destroy you.

Dad's passing hit the whole family hard, particularly Auntie Kitty, whose older brother Alfred had been killed in a car accident, leaving her as the sole survivor. I was obviously distraught, but initially I managed to carry on pretty much as normal. At least it looked that way on the outside.

Mum was exhausted from looking after him for so long, so my focus was on making sure she was coping. Meanwhile, I was still teaching at Whalley Range, in challenging circumstances, while doing my athletics and trying, unsuccessfully, to get into the senior England netball team (if you weren't playing in the London area back then, you didn't really get seen). Staying busy is a good short-term coping mechanism when you lose a loved one, but not in the long term, because you don't process your feelings.

I met Bob White, director of physical education at the University of Leicester, while competing in athletics. We got to know each other well and he ended up inviting me to work for him at Leicester, where he said I could concentrate on my sport and also get a Master's degree.

I wasn't convinced that studying for a Master's was a good idea – after all, I hadn't managed to pass a single A-level

– but Bob wasn't taking no for an answer. So in the summer of 1972, I said goodbye to my colleagues and pupils at Whalley Range, handed over the keys to my bedsit and headed back to the Midlands.

My role at Leicester wasn't well defined, but I was essentially Bob's deputy. I'm pretty sure he invented the position for me, and it involved running the undergraduate recreation programme, organising and putting on classes. I suppose you could say it was my first foray into sports administration.

I spent the first two years studying for an adult and community diploma, which felt a bit pointless to start with. It was all about community development and understanding how adults learn, and I still planned to go back to teaching in schools. But I became intrigued as to why so few young women at the university were using the sports facilities, even more so when I started reading up on the subject. Not that there was much empirical evidence out there.

A lot of theory had been written about the dissonance between the female body and the athletic body – in other words, lots of women equated being athletic (competitiveness, being muscled and sweaty) with masculinity. There were some great British female athletes in the 1960s and 1970s – Anita Lonsbrough, an Olympic swimming champion in 1960; Mary Rand and Ann Packer, who both won Olympic gold in 1964, in the long jump and 800m respectively; Mary Peters, Olympic pentathlon champion in 1972 – but they were almost otherworldly. I looked at them and thought, 'They are amazing, I'd love to be like them,' but most girls looked at them and thought, 'I'm never going to be like them – look at the muscles on them for starters!'

So I started thinking, 'How do we make physical activity more accessible? How do we shift the perception from sport being this serious business that is the preserve of a brilliant élite on the telly to sport being a fun and socially acceptable way for ordinary women to keep fit and healthy?'

I realised that to make physical activity accessible to as many people as possible, you had to understand their different motivations. And where girls and women were concerned, you had to emphasise that physical activity couldn't just make you feel better, it could make you look better. It was about trying to make physical activity and traditional notions of femininity collide.

Because people in the early 1970s weren't so celebrity-obsessed as today, I wasn't aware that fashionable people saying physical activity was great for women could be highly influential. That only became clear when the Hollywood star Jane Fonda released her 'Workout' video in the early 1980s. Suddenly, women all over the developed world were 'feeling the burn' and getting sweaty in their living rooms, and once-niche activities such as aerobics, jogging and yoga were seen as normal.

Having gained my adult and community diploma, my Master's dissertation was about understanding what inspired people to get involved in physical activity and how to build adherence to exercise. It was the kind of sports psychology stuff my Dad would have been a whizz at, and would prove to be far more useful in my career than I imagined at the time.

When I wasn't doing my paid job or studying, I was training like a demon. The hall of residence was opposite a running track, where I spent a lot of my time. I also managed to fight my way into the senior England netball team, having finally realised that I preferred competing as part of a group than as an individual.

I never felt entirely confident being out there on my own as an athlete. And when I did win, satisfying as it was, it didn't feel as uplifting as when I won as part of a team, because I wasn't able to share that special moment.

Many individual sportspeople have described the sense of hollowness after winning a major event – after winning the Open Championship, the American golfer David Duval looked at the Claret Jug and thought, 'Is that it?' – but you rarely hear sportspeople who have won as a team member talking in those terms. Indeed, it's common to hear golfers describe winning the Ryder Cup as the greatest moment of their career, despite all their individual glory.

I've met a lot of very successful individual sportspeople down the years, and they're often complex characters. No wonder, because individual sport is a lonely pursuit of excellence, and the responsibility for winning is almost all on them. And when they do win, it's impossible for anyone else to understand that feeling. Individual glory at the highest level must be a strangely isolating experience.

In contrast, when you're part of a team, responsibility is shared. And when you win as a team, you're fulfilling hopes and dreams that were never just yours: they were part of a collective, so a bond is created that never breaks. In 2022, decades after my own sporting career ended, I watched England's women's football team win the Euros and basked in the specialness of that shared moment. I wasn't part of the team, but I felt like I was. I hadn't felt that kind of overwhelming pride since playing netball for my country.

I was, and still am, very patriotic. And I'll never forget the feeling of pulling on an England shirt for the first time. It was a couple of days before the game, but I just wanted to feel it against my skin. And I thought, 'I've dreamed of this for as long as I can remember. Here I am with the red rose on my chest. This is it. I've made it.'

I won quite a few caps for England at netball, including on tours to South Africa and Jamaica. And it's telling that while I don't remember much about the games, I do remember, with great fondness, the people I toured with and the tremendous fun we had. Like the time we visited an ostrich farm and an ostrich ended up riding me, rather than the other way round.

As funny as that might sound – and it was hysterical to those who witnessed it – I always found it difficult relating those kinds of stories to anyone outside the group, because it was all about the specialness of the shared experience. As British and Irish Lions coach Ian McGeechan said in his famous 1997 tour speech, also in South Africa: 'You'll meet each other in the street in thirty years' time and there will just be a look. And you'll know just how special some days in your life are.'

After England's first game of the 2022 Euros, against Austria at Old Trafford, captain Leah Williamson explained why she'd sung the national anthem with her eyes shut. 'I thought, "There's no way I'm going to get through this if I can see my parents crying." I would have been in absolute pieces.' If Dad had been there to see me play netball for England, I would have had to do the same.

When I was first picked for England, my immediate instinct was to phone home. But Dad no longer being there, Mum picked up instead. 'I've got fantastic news,' I gushed, 'I've been selected to play for England.' 'That's wonderful, dear,' said Mum. 'Will you be home in time for tea?'

That's just the way things were back then. It wasn't that she didn't care: it was more that she didn't understand. Most women from that generation didn't understand sport, probably because they were almost expected not to.

Mum never really worked out what I did all my life, but it didn't bother me. The most important thing was that she was always there for me.

Mum carried on working after having two children, which was quite unusual in those days, but she was there every morning, and every afternoon when I got home from school. Sport might have been a mystery to her, other than the odd round of golf, but other stuff mattered greatly to her, like making sure we ate well and always had clean clothes. And not once did she ask why I was concentrating so much on sport and not doing better academically. She loved and accepted me for who I was, which meant I went to places other people feared to go and had the confidence to disrupt things once I was there.

For about a year after Dad's passing, I didn't allow myself to think about the fact that he was gone. For a while after starting at Leicester, I lived with Mum, not so much to look after her, more just to be there for her. But after moving out and into a hall of residence, I suddenly started deteriorating.

I don't know how I managed to stay standing on that tour of South Africa, let alone play netball, because I was really unwell and desperately thin. There are photos of me in my kit and I resemble a skeleton. Not a pretty sight. Shocking, actually.

Today, a lot of anorexia is driven by social media and an obsession with how people look – or are 'supposed' to look. But every individual who suffers from anorexia is different, and although people think of it as an eating disorder, it is usually linked to deep-seated anxiety, fear or some kind or an internal struggle. And while at the time I was unable to explain why I'd turned in on myself, either to loved ones or myself, later I recognised that it was about the loss of some-one who was so central to my existence: my dad.

My doctor recognised that I was suffering from anorexia, but in those days ordinary GPs didn't have a clue how to deal with it. And I can't imagine what it must have been like for Mum, watching a daughter she loved so much waste away and not being able to help her.

One thing Mum really prided herself on was giving her family great food, and here was this person who wouldn't eat anything. I was never bulimic, but I'd throw food out of windows, which must have been soul-destroying for her. She just couldn't understand why someone with so much potential seemed intent on killing herself, and while she did try to talk to me about it, I was in a complete state of denial. My sister Gill, who was away training to be an air traffic controller, would phone me and say, 'For goodness sake, stop being pathetic and get some food down you!' She wasn't being horrible: she's just very pragmatic. But if it was that simple, I'd have done it.

At Leicester, Bob White and his wife Jean, two of the loveliest people, did their best to help, which was sometimes a thankless task. Your mind, body and personality are all joined up, and when your body starts to disintegrate, so does your spirit. My body was craving food and energy, and one of the places it was looking was my nerve endings, which are home to protein. So I'd turned into a spiky, irritable, bad-tempered person who was difficult to be around.

When he could see I was really struggling, Bob would suggest we go to the golf course. I'd usually tell him I didn't have time, but he'd bundle me into his car and off we'd go to hit some balls. Bob was nowhere near as good at golf as my dad, but he looked so much like him it was spooky. At times, it was like having Dad back, which could be both a good and a bad thing.

It was when I came down with the flu that things got very serious. I was home at the time, and Mum's sister Evelyn had come to help look after me. One day, after they'd carried me to the toilet (which wasn't difficult, because there was almost nothing of me), I heard Auntie Evelyn say to Mum, 'You know she's going to die, don't you?' I remember thinking, 'Who on earth is she talking about?' It was only when I heard Mum getting very upset that I realised Auntie Evelyn was talking about me.

I kept slipping in and out of consciousness, so Mum sent for the doctor (in those days, it was normal for a family doctor to visit you at home). When he'd finished taking my vital signs, he said to me, 'I'm not sure I can help you any more. You're not listening. But you should know that you're killing your mother.' I asked him what he meant, and he replied, 'You're killing your mother with worry.' With that, he got up and left the room.

It was a while before I felt my Mum come in and sit on the end of my bed. I said to her, in barely a whisper, 'Mum, the doctor says I'm killing you,' and she started to cry, bless her. Mum hardly ever cried, so it was quite shocking when she did. She told me how hopeless she felt, that she didn't know what to do to help me, and I replied, 'Oh my good-ness. I'm so sorry.' Then I said, 'Didn't you offer me some rice pudding yesterday? Is there any left?' 'Are you sure?' said Mum, with a smile, and off she went to fetch me some.

I wasn't aware how close to death I was, and it was only when the doctor explained what I was doing to Mum that I realised I loved her more than I loved myself. That's why I always say that Mum gave birth to me twice, because by focusing on her, rather than me, I became myself again. Not that I scoffed that bowl of rice pudding and everything went back to normal, like in a Disney film. It was a slow road back to full physical and mental health. Recovering from anorexia is a physical, mental and emotional journey. There are good days and challenging days, but it is about taking things day by day.

I'm sure a psychologist would have had a field day analysing what was going on in my head, but this was the early 1970s, so I just had to work things out myself. In truth, I still don't know what I was trying to achieve, but I wasn't consciously trying to kill myself. Maybe it was a cry for help or attention. I've no doubt it had a lot to do with the fear of living without Dad, because he wasn't just my dad: he was also my friend, mentor and mind coach.

Mum and I talked about it a lot, and while she was honest about the effect my illness had on her, she never once held it against me. As I got better, the full extent of what I'd done to her started to dawn on me, and I felt terrible guilt. What an awful thing to do to someone who loves you so profoundly. But as time went on, I think we both began to view it as a special shared moment and became closer than anyone would have realised.

One of Mum's special survival weapons was her incredible sense of humour, which she had to the very end. Let me give you an example. Every year I'd take her on holiday, wherever she fancied going. One summer, we stayed in a converted lighthouse in Cornwall. She got the room at the top, right under the beacon, and I took the room below, so she could bang on the floor with her Zimmer frame if she needed me in the night. When I brought her a cup of tea on the first morning and asked if she'd slept well, she said to me, 'Not really. Some silly person was turning the light on and off all night . . .'

My anorexia also gave me a much more compassionate view of people who get into difficult situations in life.

It's easy to be critical of people with addictions, whether it's drink, drugs, cigarettes or junk food – 'Why,' people ask, 'can't they stop doing what they're doing if it's killing them?' – and there is an element of selfishness to any self-destructive behaviour. But having almost destroyed myself and come out the other side, I now understood that it was far deeper than that.

People who engage in self-destructive behaviour are not in control of themselves. Maybe they had an element of control in the beginning – when they were able to drink, take drugs, smoke or eat junk food in moderation – but at some point, those things started controlling them. And when they take charge, you're in real danger.

Empathy is understanding that even when somebody appears to be a lost cause, they can get through it with the love of another human being. In my case, my mum.

When I was a guest on *Desert Island Discs*, my final track was Diana Ross's 'Reach Out And Touch (Somebody's Hand)', because, as the second line says, my instinct is to 'make this world a better place' for other people. It's why I can't walk past anybody sitting on the street. I won't give them money, because I don't know what they're going to do with it, but I'll find a shop and buy them a hot drink and something to eat. And it's why I want people to know that if they're in difficulty, they can give me a call and I'll be there for them.

Perhaps the greatest irony of anorexia is that you need an incredibly strong will to make yourself that ill. Your whole body is screaming for food and you're choosing to deny it. But that dogged determination and wilfulness that almost killed me has held me in good stead ever since, which is why I often say to people, 'Your greatest strength is your greatest weakness, and your greatest weakness is your greatest strength.' If I could play international sport during my darkest moment, on two twigs for legs, what could I achieve when well?

Having come back from the brink, I realised how lucky I was to be the athlete I'd been and I became a lot more aware of the importance of a healthy lifestyle – eating well, exercise, things I'd taken for granted as a child.

It was three or four years before I stopped counting the calories on my plate and understanding that a bit of 'bad' food every now and again isn't necessarily a terrible thing. But now, if you ask anybody who knows me about my favourite food, they'll tell you it's chips, in a heartbeat. My local pub fries its chips in beef dripping. Twice. And I could eat them every night!!

5

Learning from the best

Remain humble and open to different ways of
working – if you stop learning, retire

In 1976, Loughborough College of Physical Education became Loughborough University's department of physical education and sports science, which meant the powers that be were obliged to admit women for the first time.

Consequently, the department was looking for its first full-time female member of staff, to provide the leadership and support for the women students. As luck would have it, Bob White was one of Loughborough's external examiners, so I'd already got to know a lot of people there and had a better sense of how things worked and what was expected of the students and staff in the department.

I'd fallen in love with the place before I even applied for the job. Everyone in tracksuits, the squeaking of trainers on gym floors and the ubiquitous smell of Deep Heat cream. Loughborough University felt like heaven designed to my exact specifications. It was a long application process, and far from easy, but I was beyond delighted when they finally offered me the job.

I'll never forget my first day, driving towards the university in my African-violet-coloured tracksuit, which is *the standard kit* at Loughborough. When the residential tower came into view, I felt goosebumps all over, and I thought, 'I cannot believe I actually work here ...'

Having parked the car, I walked with trepidation to Martin Hall common room, feeling like a child on her first day of school. And when I walked in, there were African violet tracksuits everywhere, all worn by men.

One man standing at the counter getting coffee looked very familiar. 'Gosh,' I thought, 'I know him from somewhere.' He noticed me looking at him, wandered over and said, 'Get to the right side of the corridor!' before breaking into a big grin. It was Rod Thorpe, who had been a prefect at Long Eaton Grammar School and would become my best buddy.

This being 1976, and Loughborough having never had a woman on its PE staff full-time, you might expect me to paint a picture of a sexist environment, full of men either intent on taking me down a peg or two or ignoring me completely. But it wasn't like that. Maybe, because I was still young, I didn't notice the odd bloke for whom having a woman around the place was anathema. But Rod and his colleagues made me feel right at home from the very beginning.

If anything, it was me who had a problem, because I thought I must be really special to have landed this job. I began to shed that attitude after a team-teaching session with Rod and his close friend Rex Hazeldine. Back in the common room, Rod suddenly said, 'Right, shall we start?'

'Start what?' I replied.

'We always have a debrief, say what we think about each other's teaching.'

'I don't need that.'

'OK, you go and get the coffees and me and Rex will do it.'

Off I went to get the coffees and when I returned, Rod and Rex were having a very open and forthright exchange.

The critical analysis went on for about ten minutes, until Rod finally said, 'Anyway, Rex, what are we doing this afternoon? Another coffee?'

I was very confused. They'd just had what appeared to be a big disagreement and had now switched back to being best buddies again, like someone had flicked a switch. Then Rex turned to me and said, 'Sue, remember one simple thing: if you ever stop learning, you may as well retire.'

'OK,' I replied, slightly stunned. 'Do you want to tell me what you thought of me?'

With that, Rod and Rex launched into a long and very detailed critique of my performance, which I didn't take too kindly at first. But I realised it wasn't personal: it was a professional masterclass.

Rod and Rex weren't trying to belittle me – they just wanted me to be the best I could possibly be. Because the better I was, the better our sessions would be, and the more our students would learn. I learned something really important from this exchange: the power of peer review, honest appraisal and forthright communication. Another lesson learned!

I later worked out that their initial conversation, during which they appeared to be tearing each other apart, was partly a performance for my benefit. Nevertheless, the criticism was never less than frank. And I very quickly realised that just because I was the proud owner of an African violet tracksuit, that didn't mean I'd made it.

As welcoming as the other lecturers were, they thought I was a bit of an oddball. A lot of them had been at Loughborough a long time, while I was a ball of energy, unable to hide my excitement at having got a job there. My office was directly opposite Rod's, and just sharing a cup of tea with him, both of us with our feet on the desk, chewing over the day, was thrilling to me.

Rod was the best teacher I'd ever seen. First and foremost, he loved what he was doing. Second, his students loved him. No matter how he explained things he had the students in the palm of his hand.

Rod had this great understanding of how to build practice, so that the students were never exposed to failure. It was all about small steps, so that by the end the students were doing things that looked incredibly difficult at the outset. He also found ways of including everyone in a group of varying abilities. It didn't matter if he was dealing with the most talented in the group or the least able, nobody ever felt that Rod wasn't talking to them or couldn't help them get better.

Rod and I had a set of students in two groups for tennis – definitely not one of my strengths! I went and watched Rod's sessions before teaching mine, with a view to copying him. Rod was fizzing down topspin serves and hitting the lines with topspin backhands, and I was standing there thinking, 'How on earth am I going to do that?' I listened to absolutely everything he said and made fastidious notes. When I gave them to Rod afterwards, he said, 'These are the best teaching notes I have ever had.'

When it came to my tennis session, I just demonstrated the action but did not attempt to hit the ball! Unlike Rod, I never did master topspin serves or backhands – and I wasn't a patch on him as a teacher – but I learned a huge amount just by watching him work.

In the early 1980s, Rod co-wrote a seminal work called *Teaching Games for Understanding*, which influenced how PE was taught across the globe. His co-author was another Loughborough legend, Dave Bunker, who was one of the first sports psychologists to work with a British Olympic team and supported the modern pentathlon team who won a bronze medal in 1988.

These were people who had spent years honing their craft even before arriving at Loughborough, so were experts in the proper sense of the word. There was also Derek Quant, the brilliant gymnastics coach, and the great George Gandy, who arrived at Loughborough in 1971 and quickly transformed the university's athletics programme into a world-class talent factory.

George, who sadly passed away in 2020, coached or supported some of the finest athletes Britain has ever produced, including Dave Moorcroft, Kirsty Wade, Wendy Sly, Christina Boxer, Steve Backley, Lisa Dobriskey and Paula Radcliffe. I often had to run our 'joint' sessions on my own, because George was too busy working with future record holders and Olympians.

One day, I'd laid out cones, got the students into small groups, given instructions and was ready to start my session when I noticed this skinny youth running very elegantly round the track. I shouted at him, 'Excuse me, what do you think you're doing?' And he shouted back, 'What does it look like?' I wasn't used to such impudence from Loughborough students, and shot back, 'Don't be so cheeky. This is my track, I've got a session to teach, you need to get off.'

As this youth was wandering off in a bit of a huff, one of my students said, 'Who was that?' And another student replied, 'That's Sebastian Coe . . .' Oh dear, not the best introduction to one of the greatest athletes of my time.

While I'd never seen Seb, I'd already heard a lot about him and knew he was destined for great things. Just a couple of years after our inauspicious first meeting, he broke three world records in forty-one days. And in 1980, he won gold and silver at the Moscow Olympics. His principal coach was his dad Peter, but he credited George, who was also a lecturer in biomechanics and (in)famous for his gruelling gym circuits, with making him stronger and faster.

Seb and I became firm friends in later years, but he's never stopped telling people that I'm the only person ever to throw him off a track.

Jim Greenwood was a brilliantly innovative rugby coach who'd played for Scotland and the British and Irish Lions. He was an advocate of fifteen-man 'total rugby', with forwards and backs playing as a unit and every player on the pitch interchangeable. His ideas were so influential that he earned the nickname 'Mr Rugby' in New Zealand, which is about the biggest honour imaginable.

Clive Woodward was one of his students when I was at Loughborough, and he's on record as saying he only went there because of Jim. Clive, who went on to play for England and coach them to victory in the World Cup in 2003, also says that Jim's *Total Rugby* is the only coaching book he's ever read.

One day, Jim asked if he could watch one of my netball coaching sessions. My ego still being a bit out of control, and with no knowledge of Jim's reputation, I thought to myself, 'Oh, that's nice, he wants to learn a few things.' I proceeded to do a flamboyant session, barking lots of instructions, pointing here, there and everywhere, getting the players to do exactly what I wanted them to do. Telling, telling, telling.

Afterwards, Jim asked if I wanted to come and watch him coach. The first thing that struck me was how quiet he was. He didn't shout, he didn't do much instructing. He spent most of his time watching, besides occasionally walking over to have conversations with small groups, before walking off again. And the whole time I was thinking, 'This guy's really not very good.'

In the pub afterwards, Jim asked me what I thought of his session. I told him that he needed to give more direction, and plenty more besides. Then I asked what he thought about my training session. There was a pause, before Jim muttered, 'Interesting . . .' I have since realised that when people describe something as interesting, it's not always a compliment, and it's a word that's always made me shudder since.

We did the same the following week, and this time I really pulled out all the stops. Afterwards, Jim said to me, 'I thought about what you said last week, and I've decided that it is really not my style. When you come and watch me again, come with me when I talk with those small groups and listen to what I'm saying.'

I did as he asked, and I still wasn't impressed. He'd wander over and ask questions of small groups – 'You're two points down with five minutes to go. I've set up the defence like this, what are you going to do?' – before wandering off again. Afterwards, he'd run through their decision-making with them: 'Why did you do that? What if you'd done this instead?' I was thinking, 'This guy is terrible. Why doesn't he just tell them what to do?'

In the pub, I said to him, 'You know there are books and videos to help with coaching?' I didn't know at the time that he'd written most of them. His *Total Rugby* book was considered the best of its kind.

I asked Jim what he thought of my session, and he came out with the same one-word answer: 'Interesting.' 'You said that last week,' I replied, and he said to me, 'I just want to ask you one simple question: where do you sit when the game starts?'

'I sit on the bench.'

'So who makes all the decisions on the court?'

'The players do.'

'And when do they practise that?'

Ouch.

It was less like a penny dropping and more like a brick falling on my head. It doesn't matter how well you prepare your team technically and tactically – blasting statements at them, telling, telling, telling – plans will get disrupted, so your players need to be able to work things out for themselves. They need to be nimble decision-makers, rather than programmed automatons. Plus, if there's a decent crowd watching, the players will not be able to hear you, however much you shout and scream from the sidelines.

I'd been head girl at school, senior student at Bedford, captained England Under-21s at netball, but I didn't really know what good leadership was. But that conversation with Jim, besides making me a lot more humble, taught me that leadership wasn't about being out front and shouting your head off – bouncing from place to place like a pinball, spitting out instructions, trying to dictate what should happen – it was about asking the right questions, giving the right feedback, talking to people individually, making them take responsibility, effectively encouraging them to be their own coaches.

Jim's methods were way ahead of their time and have met with resistance even in the professional era. Brian Ashton, whose philosophy is similar to Jim's, almost had a mutiny on his hands at the 2007 Rugby World Cup because his players didn't appreciate his hands-off coaching style. The irony being, when the players took control – which is what Brian wanted them to do all along – they started performing and almost won the final.

Even when England won the Rugby World Cup in 2003, some players were reluctant to give Clive Woodward too much credit. Clive believed in innovation and finding those marginal gains that we talk about in sport, but not all the players appreciated his lateral thinking.

From Jim, Clive learned the importance of thorough preparation and attention to detail, which bordered on the obsessive. He worked out a system and the people and resources necessary to make that system a reality. He brought in all sorts of different people who would have been quite unconventional at the time, such as a 'vision specialist'. And like all great head coaches, he appointed great assistant coaches. He created an élite environment in which everyone could perform to their absolute best. Clive was the ultimate facilitator and his team delivered one of England's greatest sporting victories on a world stage.

★   ★   ★

Jim and my other colleagues didn't just change my coaching style, they also had a big influence on my style of management further down the line. Good coaching, good leadership in general, is about getting the best out of people.

Ask anyone who's worked with me, and they'll tell you that I like to empower people and create an environment in which they can perform to their best. If they need some support, I'll always be there. And while I'll never tell them how to do their job, I will ask an awful lot of questions, just like Jim. My philosophy on developing people is best summed up by the words 'roots to grow and wings to fly' – feeling safe, valued and respected, but with the freedom to find your own solutions and innovate.

The first year Loughborough went co-educational, it took in twenty-eight female students. I didn't just teach them; I was in charge of the women's teams. They were all for equal opportunities, quite rightly, and feisty, but I thought the best way of changing attitudes to women was by doing rather than talking. I thought that by showing how proud they were to represent Loughborough, they'd make everyone else at the university proud of them.

Early in our first term together, I got them all in a room and said, 'Look, some men here think we're going to be a complete disaster. They think we're going to drag down standards. But you know what? It's going to be the complete opposite. We're actually going to be the very best – the best at netball, the best at hockey, the best academically. Let's do this!'

That's exactly what happened, because they were an incredibly talented group of women who could turn their hand to anything. The netball and hockey teams couldn't stop winning, but the event that summed those women up best was a British Universities Athletics Championship in 1976.

On the way there, I was running up and down the bus telling each student what event they'd be competing in: 'You're doing the javelin, you're doing the high jump, you're doing the 800m . . .' Some of them had never competed in those events before, and I remember saying to the poor girl I'd roped in to do the 800m, 'Don't worry, just remember not to stop after the first lap and keep going to the end, no matter what.' The young woman I asked to do the hurdles fell several times but valiantly got up and carried on to the finish line. A testimony to their grit, determination and desire to achieve. The whole group were willing to do absolutely anything I asked them – and ended up winning the overall title.

As gifted as those women were, they also worked like demons. Early in my tenure, I said to the netball team, 'If you just want to do the timetabled training, you can. But I'm going to be in the gym at seven every morning, and if you want to join me, you can.' Two of them turned up on the first day, then five or six on the second. But within a week, they were all coming. And because I made it fun, with varied circuits and music, we had an absolutely brilliant time.

They also proved a point in lectures, where they were soon outgunning the boys academically, probably because they worked harder. They were determined to show that they were worthy of respect in every way.

The more the female students impressed, the less I felt like the token woman at Loughborough. I was just Sue and got on famously with almost all the male lecturers. One of the loveliest was Alan Guy, who was everything that Bob White had been to me at Leicester. Alan was a lecturer rather than a coach (an excellent one, I should add), but he took a huge interest in everything I did. He'd come to my netball games with his daughter, and I could always go to him if I was struggling with something. He was a very kind, clever man who provided the emotional support and philosophical advice to go with all the practical lessons I was learning from the best of the Loughborough line-up. Mentors are so important at every stage of our lives.

Before Loughborough, I'd understood my own search for sporting excellence, but I hadn't seen a brand and a system that was totally geared to excellence.

I had a premier job in an élite environment with élite people and I'd fallen in love with coaching, to the extent that I appreciated it more than performing myself. Everyone assumed I'd be at Loughborough for the next forty years. It was wonderful and I adored it — but it didn't satisfy something in me. All the time I was working with those wonderful young women, winning everything in sight, I never forgot class 4O at Whalley Range High School.

I had been at Loughborough for four years when a man called Peter Warburton, who was a senior regional officer for the East Midlands Sports Council, popped into the university and started talking to me about how we could use sport as a vehicle for social change. Then he dropped the bombshell that he had a job vacancy that needed filling, which involved working with disadvantaged communities, people who had been written off as unreachable and unchangeable – the elderly, the disabled, mothers in high-rise buildings, the unemployed, kids from inner-city estates and deprived rural areas.

There I was, ensconced in excellence at Loughborough, loving every minute of it, and now I had the option of working with people who didn't do sport at all. Most sane people would have rejected the offer in a heartbeat. But the itch had become inflamed and desperately needed scratching. As cornily idealistic as it sounds, I had to go and change some lives.

6

The power of connection

Building alliances and partnerships can help you
reach much further than you can ever reach alone

My Loughborough colleagues all thought I'd lost my mind.
Rod sat me down, like a concerned uncle with a child who
was in danger of going off the rails, and said, 'What are you
doing? I think you're making a terrible mistake.'

'I know you do,' I replied. 'Everyone here does. But something is drawing me back to the inner-city mission.'

'Can't you just take a bit of leave, get it off your chest and
come back?'

'No. I can't explain why, but I have to go and do it. And
not look back.'

I was helping to change lives at Loughborough, but my
students were already on an upward trajectory. Few would
end up playing sport for a living (even someone as talented as
Clive, because rugby union was still amateur back then), but
they'd become PE teachers, sports scientists, psychologists or

something else entirely (Seb studied economics and history, which was something to fall back on if his athletics career didn't pan out as expected).

I suppose I felt that I was being a little bit self-indulgent – Loughborough was such a lovely, comfortable existence. I couldn't stop thinking about the dormant potential I'd awoken in Manchester – and all the potential that remained untapped. Could I do things better? Could I do things on a larger scale? I knew that I couldn't expect the people I would be working with to go on to be élite sportspeople, but hoped that, through sport, I might be able to change their lives for the better.

Sporting excellence still fascinated me intellectually (when I took on the new job I continued coaching athletics and East Midlands netball, and was defence assistant coach for the England team), but my heart was in using sport to make the world a better place. I'd spend my whole career switching between those two things – from Whalley Range to Leicester, from Loughborough to the inner cities, and so it went on.

On paper, I was well suited to my new position with the East Midlands Sports Council. I had my adult and community diploma from Leicester University, as well as my Master's dissertation, and I'd worked with disadvantaged children at Whalley Range High School. But I soon realised that while I had a good idea of how to change the lives of people I was in direct contact with, I had no idea how to change lots of lives via a bigger system. I still didn't really know what sport development was.

Whether it was working in Hyson Green in Nottingham, the Saffron Lane estate in Leicester, deprived rural areas in Derbyshire and Lincolnshire, it was never less than challenging. During the four years I was there – from 1979 to 1983 – I got a lot of things wrong, but that's one of the best ways of learning. And I learned so much about the power of sport to change lives and improve society.

When I first arrived at Loughborough, I was lucky to be surrounded by people who knew exactly what they were doing, which rubbed off on me (at least after my humility kicked in). Mercifully, it was the same in the inner cities.

Jim Teatum was the first-ever community police officer in Leicester and some of the things I saw him achieve were incredible. I worked with him around the time of the 1981 riots, which affected many cities and towns in the East Midlands. He was dealing with youngsters who were angry and aggressive – and had every right to be. Many of them were Black and Asian young people who didn't feel part of British society, but Jim could get through to them. They could feel his love and compassion, and get that he genuinely wanted to make their lives better.

I witnessed Jim change some of the toughest, worst-behaved kids in Leicester into confident, proud young men with respect for themselves and other people. I felt so privileged to work alongside Jim – and there were plenty of others like him, people who understood the challenges of people's lives and who were doing their very best to improve them.

Jim said to me one day, 'Sue, I want to put on a course to train young men to be leaders, but I don't know who to bring in.' I replied, 'I've got some people I think can help,' before jumping in my car and heading back to Loughborough. Over coffee in the common room, I said to Rod, Rex and Dave, 'What do you do on Saturday mornings?' Their answers ranged from 'Preparing for matches' to 'Shopping'!

'Well,' I said, 'I've got something a lot more interesting for you.'

'What are you on about?'

'For the next six Saturdays, I want you to come to this hall in Leicester and teach leadership to a group of young men for a couple of hours.'

'You're joking?'

'No.'

'Is there any money in it?'

'No.'

'Oh, Sue . . .'

'Come on, you can do it.'

'Oh, go on then . . .'

Sure enough, all three of my superstars turned up the following Saturday, resplendent in their African-violet tracksuits and spotless white trainers. They'd also taken the time to write a leadership programme, which formed the basis of the very successful Central Council of Physical Recreation (now the Sport and Recreation Alliance) leadership programme. And remember: they were doing all this for no monetary reward.

The young men, mostly Rastafarians, arrived an hour late, which annoyed the Loughborough team – the first clear message that these young men were not Loughborough students. Rod's approach was not to chastise them, so he simply said, 'Sorry you missed the first hour, that was the best part. Never mind, we'll move on ...'

It was an inauspicious start, but it blossomed into something magical. The participants turned up earlier the second week and really started responding. For the final session, Jim brought along some younger people for the trainee leaders to work with. And I spent most of the two hours laughing my head off in the corner, because the young men had morphed into mini-versions of Rod, Rex and Dave. In the end, I said to them, 'You have got to stand back and have a look at this ...'

Three of them were waving their arms around and doing everything at 100mph, just like Rex. Three of them were taking a more gentle, hands-off approach, just like Rod. And the other three were explaining things very methodically, just like Dave. The young men had modelled themselves on the personality that best fitted them, and it demonstrated that there are many different ways of leading, all equally valid. I've got a lovely picture of the four of us watching those young men, with big smiles on our faces. It captures the joy of changing lives through sport.

Many of the people I was trying to engage with were very isolated, physically and mentally. They also had narrow horizons, because they'd come through an education system that had not drawn out the best in them or shown them what was possible.

Some of the elderly people I interacted with were vibrant, despite their straitened circumstances, but some had lost all purpose. They couldn't afford to do much, if anything, or were too frightened to leave their homes, because they had lost confidence. Would sport solve all their problems? Of course not: I was an idealist, but I wasn't delusional. But I was convinced that even a bit of activity a week could make a difference. Just turning up requires effort, but once you're there, you're socialising and hopefully making friends.

Physical activity isn't just about keeping fit; it's also about the mental and spiritual benefits. Not being able to exercise has always adversely affected my mental equilibrium. Even now, if I can't give the dogs a good walk for three or four days in a row, I get fidgety and cranky. So I was beginning to understand what it must have been like for those people living in high-rises, unable to exercise because they were looking after babies and small children or caring for a wife or husband. They felt trapped, and I spent a lot of time feeling like I was trying to find them in the dark, armed only with a small torch. And while I could show them where the exit was, I couldn't make them follow me.

A key thing I learned during my time working in the inner cities was that connecting people and ideas was often the best way to solve a problem. In Nottingham, there was an amazing woman called Madge Baranek from the Keep

Fit Association, who had trained with the famous choreographer Rudolf Laban in the 1960s. Madge's energy and enthusiasm were daunting – everybody tried to hide whenever she came into our office, because she wasn't great at taking no for an answer. But when she came in search of money for a keep-fit course for the over-fifties – and explained that she'd trained lots of keep-fit teachers but couldn't find any over-fifties for them to work with – I advised her to apply for a grant and logged our conversation in my mind. As my dad used to say to me: 'Every person you speak to has something worth hearing. So listen and bank it.'

A month or so later, I was due to do an introductory sports event in Bulwell, a few miles north of Nottingham. Somebody put posters up around the town – SPORTS SESSIONS FOR THE OVER-50s – and on the scheduled day, I turned up bright and early at Bulwell Community Centre, hoping at least a handful of people might show up. But having set up some table-tennis tables and a badminton court, I spent the next hour standing on my own in this draughty hall, imagining the people of Bulwell looking at my posters and scoffing, 'Who is this lunatic?' 'Forlorn' doesn't even begin to describe the scene. It was like my first lesson with class 4O all over again.

As I was packing everything up, people started trickling in, and I thought to myself, 'Did I write the wrong time on the posters?' Alas, I hadn't got the wrong time: they were arriving for their weekly lunch club.

These people, all middle-aged, clearly all knew each other, and some of them were carrying more weight than was healthy. I remember thinking what a shame it was that I couldn't get them to do some activity. Then something in my brain clicked: 'Madge! Maybe she could do something with this group?'

I phoned Madge as soon as I got back to the office: 'You know these keep-fit courses you do for the over-fifties? Could you come and do one for me?'

The following week, Madge blew into the community centre like a whirlwind, and within ten minutes, she had them holding onto their chairs, swaying from side to side and swinging their legs, some simultaneously eating cake and drinking tea. While that was going on, I was setting up the table-tennis tables and badminton court. And once lunch/keep fit was over, about half of them stuck around for a fun session. It was wonderful to watch them enjoying themselves, be that laughing their heads off or getting competitive. I remember one woman saying to me, 'I haven't hit a ball since I was a child.'

Everyone was a winner – me, Madge and, most importantly, the people who took part in the session. Then it dawned on me: 'I wonder how many people attend lunch clubs in Nottinghamshire?'

I arranged a meeting with Madge and the organisers of these lunch clubs and floated the idea of putting a keep-fit teacher and some sports equipment into every one of them. They all thought that was a great idea, so that's exactly what we did. And those clubs lasted for many years.

That, for me, was proper sustainable sports development. By connecting things that didn't appear to have anything in common, I'd made something happen that benefited individuals and the community they lived in. If only for two hours every week, the world of the lunch club attendees became bigger, their community became tighter, they got some exercise, and they had some fun. We did the same for mums and children, combining a crèche with aerobics and coffee. In truth, it was just caring for human beings and providing them with opportunities to enrich their daily lives.

But for all the little victories, I also made so many mistakes, some of which make me cringe to this day. Like the time I was working with a group of young men with West Indian heritage and turned up with a load of cricket kit. This being the 1980s, the West Indies were kings of cricket and the game was still a big deal in Caribbean communities in England, so I thought these young men would be into it. But as it turned out, all they wanted to do was play basketball. Instead of asking, I'd lazily relied on assumptions and stereotypes.

It was also the first time I'd spent any time around people with disabilities, and I started out by being typically patronising. I'd speak to adults in wheelchairs as if they were children, thinking I was being compassionate.

I got to know a guy called John who used a wheelchair, and one day he picked me up in his car. When we arrived at our destination, I said to him, 'Can I help you with your wheelchair?' and he gave me a death stare.

'Can I just stop you there?' he said. 'You are a real pain.'

'I'm so sorry,' I said. 'What have I done?'

'I'm a human being, treat me like one. I have a disability, but you don't need to overcompensate. Just talk to me like you would anyone else.'

I cried that night, but I'd learned another important lesson.

Over the coming years, I worked with a brilliant man called Dr Swanton, who ran rehab day centres all over the East Midlands, and I got better and better at interacting with people with disabilities. Dr Swanton taught me to communicate with them empathetically but not in a degrading manner, just as Jim Teatum had taught me to communicate empathetically with people with addictions and criminal records. These people had certain challenges in their lives, but, as John had made clear to me, they were still human beings.

I loved my time working in the inner cities, but I can't say it was always enjoyable, because the challenges were so great. When something good happened, the rewards were immense, which kept me ploughing on, but I came crashing down to earth plenty of times. Luckily, I'd grown sturdy roots over many years, having been nurtured by some remarkable people.

My philosophy of roots to grow and wings to fly was tested to its limit. If your roots are deep and secure, it doesn't matter if you crash – it's just another lesson learned, and you can try again, this time doing things differently.

I'd been able to demonstrate that physical activity could spread hope and happiness even in difficult circumstances, and my appetite for changing lives through sport hadn't been sated. However, when the Sports Council set up a coach development agency, Peter Warburton, who was a keen volleyball coach and loved chatting to me about it, suggested I apply for the role of CEO.

I had never stopped thinking of myself as a coach; having learned from the best I had developed an interest in how we trained and developed coaches. I did not get the CEO's job but I was offered the role of deputy. It was the continuation of the peculiar zigzagging journey that has been my career.

Calling me deputy CEO was a bit grand because there were only three of us at the National Coaching Foundation (NCF), as the agency was called, working out of a semi-detached house in Leeds. The CEO was Nick Whitehead, who won a bronze medal in the 4 x 100m relay at the 1960 Olympics and taught PE at the City of Leeds and Carnegie College. And our secretary was Jean Vorderman, mother of TV's Carol, who was worth her weight in gold.

The plan was for the Sports Council to fund the NCF for three years. If it worked, it would carry on. If it didn't, it would be dismantled. Nick was more involved with the political side of things, while I spent the first eighteen months building what I called a market stall of resources and courses, consisting of five tiers, from introductory packs for the beginner coach through to individually designed modules for élite coaches.

Frank Dick, who was director of coaching for British Athletics, had already embraced sports science (he'd studied the East German system and realised they weren't just successful because of doping), but most British coaches in 1984 were fixated on technique and tactics, while believing that things like psychology, biomechanics and conditioning were not central to the education of coaches. Many of them found additional knowledge and support along the way but there was no systematic way of embedding the 'ologies', and there was great deal of cynicism and fear in the face of something different.

One of the NCF's main aims was to get more coaches thinking like Frank. To that end, I took all the 'ologies' and broke them into bite-sized chunks. I ended up with a set of six introductory packs for beginner coaches looking at planning, fitness, working with young people, motivation and so on, many of them authored by my Loughborough colleagues! But at the top end, there were more advanced courses on endurance, aerobic and anaerobic training, nutrition, rehydration and mental preparation – fine-tuning the athlete to achieve their potential.

The introductory study packs were quickly written and published, but the courses at the higher levels required a different approach. I went to Loughborough, Birmingham University and the Carnegie College of PE in Leeds and asked colleagues if they'd write some modules for me – for nothing, of course. However, I also told them that they could deliver our courses on their premises, and that they'd be able to keep all the money they brought in. They all delivered, brilliantly, and I ended up with twenty modules written by some of the best sports-science brains in the country, being taught at fourteen universities which we named National Coaching Centres. Thousands of coaches across all the major sports attended the courses, and governing bodies started to adopt the modules into their coach-development programmes.

Initially, selling those ideas to élite coaches was a very difficult task. I visited all the national coaches in each sport to 'persuade' them to adopt the modules but was not always greeted warmly!

The first British Association of National Coaches Conference I attended was a less than positive experience. I had to give a talk to all the coaching directors in an auditorium, and every one of them was male, except for Penny Chuter from rowing. I explained how I thought there were different ways of looking at coaching, with the athlete at the centre and sports science to the fore, not just technique and tactics, and they all sat there with their arms folded, faces like thunder. To say it was intimidating would be an understatement. I felt like I was singing completely out of tune.

I have been in that situation many times since and eventually learned to steel myself, recognise when I was not connecting and be brave enough to change tack. But on that occasion, I was too scared to go off script and felt very inadequate. And when I finished talking, most of the arms stayed folded and there was the tiniest ripple of applause. 'Thank you all very much,' I said. 'I'll keep working to understand how I can present this better in the future.' With that, I scuttled off the stage, I can laugh about it now — but I wasn't laughing then.

We did make progress over time, and a number of National Governing Bodies (NGBs) adopted the modules and became advocates with their colleagues. However, there were still those who thought I was just someone who had read too many books and had the audacity to tell them how to coach. I could understand someone like Frank Dick's irritation, because he was already miles ahead in his thinking. Frank and I had many challenging discussions, but through those forthright conversations we developed a strong mutual respect, and he remains a close colleague to this day.

I had one very brief meeting with Charles Hughes, who was director of coaching for the Football Association. Charles was an advocate of direct football, trying to score goals with as few passes as possible, which is in complete contrast to the modern game. And while I didn't think I'd persuade Charles to change his philosophy, I hoped he'd at least be open to hearing one or two new ideas. I was wrong! I was given a short audience with him in which he made it very clear I had nothing to offer and despatched me from his office quickly. I stood on the pavement outside the building, reflecting that I had to find a different approach if I was going to make headway in some of the bigger sports. Perhaps I needed to win over people further down the chain of command to build relationships and develop trust.

Charles had been top of the tree for a long time and was not going to take advice from me. As I had already learned, I was not going to be able to tell people what they needed: I was going to have to ask questions, listen and be agile enough to come up with solutions.

I still got knocked back and flattened in plenty of meetings, but a few of the coaching directors were good enough to take me under their wing, like Jim Greenwood had done at Loughborough. They saw me as someone trying really hard to do the right thing, even though they realised that I was disrupting years of traditional thinking.

Judo's director of coaching was Geoff Gleeson, who had been in his role for twenty-five years. Geoff would often say to me, 'You don't understand what coaching is – all the resources you are producing are about the *science* of coaching. I'm talking about the *art* of coaching.'

Geoff invited me down to London one day and took me to an art gallery. He wandered around in his flowing cape and big hat (as well as being very cultured, Geoff was quite eccentric), with me trailing behind, and suddenly stopped in front of a big mural.

'What do you think of that?' he said.

'Have they put it the right way up?' I replied.

'You're a Philistine. Look at it properly. Take in all the blues, take in all the yellows . . .'

I looked at the mural for a few minutes and I concluded it was lovely, but I still couldn't understand why Geoff had brought me there.

'Is there any point to this, Geoffrey?' I asked.

'Yes. I'm going to buy you a coffee and tell you all about it.'

Having sat ourselves down in the gallery coffee shop, Geoff started explaining himself.

'Sue, every artist starts with a paintbrush and a palette of paints. They choose to work in oils or watercolours. And there's a science to tools and materials. But what you looked at wasn't science, that was art.'

'Keep going.'

'Sue, great artists have the same scientific knowledge as everyone else. They use the same tools and materials as everyone else. But they have a personal way of expressing themselves. And that's what you're failing to see.'

Later, when Geoff invited me to his house, I couldn't find a chair to sit on, because his living room was full of newspapers, piled almost up to the ceiling. From his house, we walked through a wood to his local pub, where I quizzed him on the history of coaching in British judo.

I'd noticed that the philosophy in judo had abruptly changed over the years, rather than evolving smoothly. It was one way in the 1960s, different in the 1970s, and different again in the 1980s. It didn't make sense to me.

When I asked Geoff if the sudden changes were the result of research that had been done, he looked at me like I was mad, before replying, 'No, it simply depends on the individual writing them, and their own philosophy of the sport. That is how it works.'

As much as I loved Geoff and his philosophy of coaching, it became clear that what was needed across many sports was a more rigorous coach development framework based on insights and research in human development. The NCF did not want every coach to be the same, but there needed to be a foundation on which each individual coach could build. While Britain had some success in judo (Neil Adams was a European and world champion who also won two Olympic silver medals in 1980 and 1984), there was no understanding that while a focus on technique and tactics might produce one-off success, it had its limitations. Long-term consistent success would only be achieved when we could prepare the body and mind of each player to the highest level as well as giving them the techniques and tactics to overcome their opposition.

How much better might Britain be at sport if coaches took a more scientific approach? If instead of viewing scientific knowledge with suspicion, they embraced it and locked it into their sport? The knowledge was out there, in all corners of the globe. You just had to look for it – and have an open mind.

I went to Canada to see a man called Geoff Gowan, who had taught athletics at Loughborough in the 1960s but was now running the Canadian equivalent of the NCF (he had been unable to get people to listen to his ideas in the UK). One of Geoff's tutors gave a great talk on nutrition, all about carbohydrates, proteins and energy levels, and afterwards I asked some other attendees how the talk might affect their thinking around pre-match meals. They all looked at me with blank faces, which told me everything I needed to know. They now had the knowledge, but they either didn't want to apply it or didn't know how, so their athletes would continue to eat traditional pre-match food.

But there were encouraging signs that the messaging was starting to get through. One day, I returned to Loughborough to watch Clyde Williams deliver one of our courses, and during the four hours I could see people in the room experiencing multiple light-bulb moments.

Clyde was the founding chairman of the British Association of Sports Sciences and had an amazing knack of making science sound simple. Before that day, many of these coaches had never really appreciated the difference between aerobic and anaerobic exercise; as Clyde explained it in a language that coaches could grasp it all became clear. Halfway through, a cycling coach from Hull whispered to me, 'This guy is a genius. I'd read so many books and not understood, but I do now.'

There were coaches from lots of different sports on Clyde's course, and I'd like to think that more than a few went away better informed and ready to rethink their approach.

Did everything work well? No. But we did disrupt a mindset. Before the NCF, most coaching was purely focused on tactics and technique. But today, we take it for granted that sports science is fully integrated into élite sport.

After eighteen months in the job, Nick Whitehead left to become the Deputy Chief Executive of the Sports Council for Wales. Following an interview, I went to meet the chief executive of Sport England who told me they would be closing the NCF down in another eighteen months, because it didn't seem to be making the progress they had expected. Then he said, 'The CEO job is yours if you want it.' I didn't know whether to be happy or slightly insulted.

'Can I ask you something?' I said.

'Go ahead.'

'If at the end of the next eighteen months the NCF is financially independent, will you still shut it down? Or will you leave me to get on with it?'

'That's impossible – you will not be able to make that happen,' he said.

'Sorry, but you haven't answered my question.'

'No, we won't shut it down. But what you're proposing is not possible.'

All the way back on the train from London to Leeds my mind was buzzing; how could I generate income?

I popped in to see our secretary, Jean, on my way home.

'Have you got the job?' she said.

'Yes. But we've got to find all our own money or we will close down in eighteen months.'

'How are we going to do that?'

'No idea. But we will find a way!'

7

Relationships are key

*It takes a lot of work to build trust and develop
mutual respect with people but that is the basis
on which great relationships are made*

Rainer Martens was a professor of kinesiology (the study of human body movement) at the University of Illinois when he founded a company called Human Kinetics in the mid-1970s, with a view to selling books on physical education and sport. His was a remarkable story of someone who wrote a paper on the importance of psychology in élite sport that nobody was interested in publishing ... so he decided to do it himself.

By the mid-1980s, Rainer had established himself as a world-renowned coach educator, and his books had sold in sufficient numbers to allow him to leave the University of Illinois and commit to his company full time (his book *Successful Coaching* has sold more than a million copies, and Human Kinetics remains the biggest publisher of physical education resources in the world).

I met Rainer at a pre-Olympic congress, where he gave a brilliant talk. (The only problem was that I had to follow him, and I felt rather like a poor support act!) Afterwards, I asked him if it was possible to teach the *art* of coaching, and he maintained that you could, if you built it into the way that you trained coaches. According to Rainer, you needed to ask the right questions, not tell coaches how to do things, because if you tried to tell them, you would remove their ownership and replace it with yours. In effect, you'd stop them expressing themselves and finding the creativity that Geoff Gleeson had been talking about. It is the same in management, and it's what so many managers get wrong. They think they must instruct and tell rather than question and empower.

Rainer had a lot to teach people about a lot of things, but in 1985, with the NCF at risk of going under, I was mainly interested in his lessons in publishing. Having written all these introductory study packs, I decided to start selling them at £1.50 each. Jean made me a poster that said, 'BUY ALL SIX FOR £9', and I looked at it and said, 'Jean, that's still £1.50 a pack.' (Remember, Jean was the mother of Carol Vorderman, famous as the maths whizz on Channel 4's *Countdown*!)

We plastered these posters far and wide, and every Saturday, Jean, Carol, Maureen the cleaner and I would box the packs up, take them to the post office, then go to a local fish and chip restaurant for lunch. We weren't going to be rivalling Human Kinetics any time soon, but it was a start.

When it came to getting sponsorship, I thought I could go in, sell my passion and someone would write me a cheque. But I learned that I wasn't just selling to potential sponsors, I was actually buying *and* selling, which meant first finding out what they wanted before jumping headlong into my pitch. And it worked. After a while, people were sponsoring all sorts of things for us, including cars.

I didn't learn how to fund-raise from any books: I learned quickly, by trial and error – lots of errors. There's a lot to be said for that. Much of what I've done during my career resulted from being forced into difficult situations and simply doing what I had to do to escape them. In the case of the NCF, when we reached the end of our three-year experiment, we were self-sufficient, which meant we weren't going to be closed down and could carry on working as an independent entity.

I'm not entirely motivated by proving people wrong, but if I believe in a cause I'm going to fight for its survival tooth and nail. I suppose you could say I have a missionary zeal. So it wasn't a case of, 'You are not going to shut *me* down,' it was, 'You are not going to shut *this organisation* down.' It was just too important for sport in this country.

The NCF was the beginning of the transformation of the coaching system in the UK. As our reputation grew, we were asked to take on an additional role. Bill Slater, a wonderful man and deputy CEO of Sport England, asked if we could create a sports-science support programme for governing bodies. I said yes – and then worked out how to do it! My colleague Dr Sarah Rowell, a British former long-distance runner, had joined us at the NCF and I invited her to take on this challenge. She met with governing bodies to determine their specific sports-science research needs. She then matched them to members of the British Association of Sport and Exercise Science and provided monitoring and support throughout the programmes. It was an outstanding success, and sports began to recognise the performance value of applied science.

By the 1990s, the NCF was flying, and in a delicious irony, the Sports Council's deputy chairman Allan Patmore called us the organisation's 'jewel in the crown', which was some turnaround. A few years earlier, they'd wanted to close us down. If you'd asked me at the time, I wouldn't have been able to tell you how we made the NCF a success. It just kind of happened, and it had a lot more to do with the basic building of relationships than any genius on my part.

I recall a meeting in 1990 with Robert Atkins, who was Minister for Sport. He had spent all day meeting representatives from dozens of British sports organisations, all wanting money, and I was last on the list. When I walked into his office, he looked at his watch. I said, 'Has it been a long day, minister?' and he sighed and reeled off all the people he'd met, getting some of the acronyms wrong, which was hardly surprising. When he told me I only had a few minutes, I replied, 'I bet you're tired of listening to people, so why don't we reverse it. In those few minutes, why don't you tell me what *you* want to achieve as Minister for Sport? What do you want to be known for? What difference do you want to make?' He leaned back in his chair, thought for a moment, and said, 'I want to improve coaching and sport for young people in state schools.'

Those few minutes turned into an hour, during which time he mostly talked and I asked lots of questions and listened. When he was finished outlining his ambition, I told him the NCF would be delighted to design a scheme and run it for him.

The minister departed with the words, 'I might come back to you,' which didn't fill me with much confidence. And a couple of months later, having heard nothing from him, I discovered he was being moved to another department.

I thought that might be that, but I was in the office one day when the phone rang. I remember Jean shouting upstairs, 'Sue, it's the minister,' and me shouting back, 'You mean the minister's office.' 'No,' replied Jean, 'I mean the *actual* minister . . .'

The minister asked if I'd worked out the scheme and if I could get it to him within two hours. Then he told me that in the move to the new department he had unearthed one million pounds, but we needed to act quickly to secure the money. I had worked out the scheme in my head – coaches working at different levels, schools linking with governing bodies – but I hadn't written anything down. However, when one million pounds is on offer, you work fast.

The minister wanted it to be called 'Coaching Champions',

but I wanted it to be more inclusive (not every young person will become a champion) and preferred 'Champion Coaching'. We argued about the title for some time but in the end Champion Coaching was born ... All I had to do now was find someone to run it! That was one of my first real forays into politics, and what a brilliant concept Champion Coaching turned out to be.

On one of my many visits to Human Kinetics I met Katie Donovan — she had been an athletic director and was leading the American Coaching Effectiveness Programme across the USA for Rainer. She had extensive experience of after-school sport and coach education so was the perfect person to lead this new programme. I also recruited a talented sports development officer from Nottinghamshire local authority, Steve Grainger. He had a great reputation for turning concepts into something concrete and putting them on the ground effectively. Throughout my journey I have kept an eye out for good people because I believe the right people can make amazing things happen — and these two were an incredible combination. Both were high-energy, full of great ideas and committed to excellence.

In 1991, we rolled out Champion Coaching in twenty-four local authorities. Steve would drive all over the country handing out our newly designed coach education resources (every time he opened his boot, there would be red, green and blue boxes everywhere — he's probably still got hundreds of them in his garage!). We worked with the governing bodies to recruit suitable coaches who delivered after-school coaching sessions for eleven-to-fourteen-year-olds, using the materials we'd developed (much of it written by Dave Haskins, another member of the team and one of the country's foremost authors in sports development resources).

Katie had driven the programme brilliantly, and by the second year we had forty-four local authorities on board, including in Wales and Northern Ireland. We had also expanded the number of sports on offer to sixteen, ranging from football to orienteering.

We had started training new coaches, and in some of those areas we had handed over responsibility for the running of the scheme to local managers. Champion Coaching was a brilliant example of what can be achieved when you bring coaches (qualified and voluntary), teachers and parents together for the benefit of young people. The scheme was, without doubt, one of the biggest successes of the NCF and made a massive difference to school sport.

We recognised that we were now generating a large number of resources and publications as a result of Champion Coaching and the prolific brilliance of Penny Crisfield, our Education Director. So we took the decision to set up a wholly owned trading subsidiary – Coachwise – and acquired a warehouse! Somehow, I'd become a businesswoman.

Unfortunately for us Robert Atkins moved on and, as is often the way in politics, the next minister had his own ideas and had no interest in keeping the scheme going.

But just as the government funding was running out, I got a call from Olympic swimming champion Duncan Goodhew, who told me about a very rich man in London who was looking for a youth project to invest in over a number of years. That sounded more than intriguing, so off I went to meet him.

Sir John Beckwith was very different from me. Educated at Harrow, he went on to establish one of the country's largest real-estate companies with his brother Peter, before branching out into the financial world – insurance broking, private investment, venture capitalism, you name it.

I met Sir John at an expensive restaurant in London and we hit it off immediately, despite seemingly not having much in common. Sir John started by telling me a story: he was driving home from the office one day when he saw some teenagers fighting in the street. He said to me, 'We've got to get these kids playing sport instead of getting up to no good on the streets.' At the very basic level, John's philosophy was the same as mine: we both wanted to use physical activity and sport to change lives for the better.

Sir John asked what I'd do if he gave me one million pounds, and I outlined a series of programmes covering different age groups (the programme for eleven-to-fourteen-year-olds was essentially Champion Coaching). John loved it, and before we had even finished lunch, he offered me the money.

'Wow,' I said. 'The whole one million?'

'Yes. But you've got to come and work for me.'

'No, no. I thought you wanted to give the money to the NCF.'

'No. I want to set up something new: the Youth Sport Trust.'

'Sorry, Sir John, I can't come and work for you. I've spent ten years building up the NCF – I don't want to start all over again.'

I'd travelled to London without any intention of working for Sir John Beckwith. But he wasn't just very rich, he was also very persuasive. So, while I walked away from that lunch with a million pounds and a dream of transforming school sport and PE, he walked away with me and my blueprint, which I'd scribbled on a napkin (probably a very expensive one).

My NCF farewell event was very emotional. I'd put so much energy and hard work into that organisation, and by the time I left to set up the Youth Sport Trust (YST), it had something like two hundred employees (the NCF later became UK Coaching, which is still in existence today). But I've never been one to look back, even when the immediate future doesn't look that promising.

I managed to persuade Loughborough University to give me a room rent-free, which was very good of them. Alas, it was small, with a well-used carpet and Blu-Tack all over the walls. The YST's first day of operation was 1 May 1995, and I had appointed one employee, Mandy Bradley, as my office manager. As she walked in, she said, 'When you said we were starting afresh, I didn't quite appreciate exactly how "afresh" you meant . . .'

Mandy was a terrific person to have alongside me – she was practical, hardworking, and not afraid to turn her hand to anything. She had brought tea, coffee, biscuits, cake and a kettle, and after a quick brew, we got to work. Up came the carpet, off came the Blu-Tack and Mandy's husband Jason came and painted the walls. Jason and I then headed to the second-hand furniture store and picked up two desks and two chairs, and by the time we had returned, Mandy had the phones up and running.

I'd asked Sir John to start us off with £250,000, rather than give me the full million in one go, and one of the first things I did was recruit Steve Grainger again, this time from the NCF. Rod Thorpe had a young PhD student, Ben Tan, working with him and they had been writing some really interesting material for primary schools, and we got to work adapting it for our purposes.

The blueprint I'd written on a napkin ended up being called the 'TOPs' programmes. There was TOP Tots (for pre-school children); TOP Play (for the first two years of primary, when it's mainly about developing movement literacy – competence to move easily – run, jump, throw); and TOP Sport (mini-sports developed with the NGBs – small-sided football, tag rugby, Kwik cricket, short tennis, netball etc. for the later years of primary). Champion Coaching became TOP Club for eleven-to-fourteen-year-olds (the NCF had run out of money to fund Champion Coaching) and TOP Link for fourteen-to-eighteen-year-olds, a leadership programme to train secondary-school pupils to work with primary-school children. Something for everyone!

We knew we had to incentivise in-service training for the primary teachers as recruitment on similar courses had not been well attended. So we developed the idea of a big blue bag of child-friendly equipment – something many schools did not have – to give to every school who enrolled teachers on the TOPs training. Our only challenge was that this was going to cost over ten million pounds! I started talking to the Lottery unit at Sport England (the National Lottery had been established in 1994 and Sport England were the distributors for sports projects), but they only funded capital programmes at that time and equipment did not qualify. However, they were looking for an impact project nationally and I eventually persuaded them that TOPs was the answer!

The equipment was made by a company called Davies Sports in Nottingham, run by a wonderful man called Phil Isherwood, who bought into the mission and thought we were going to change the world. I said to Phil, 'I don't know what colours kids like, and whether those colours change as they get older,' and he ended up taking a great big Davies van around to different schools in his area, full of every bit of equipment in every colour you could think of, and letting the kids pick out the stuff that looked the most appealing.

Along with the sports equipment was a set of resource cards for teachers, with some helpful guidance to ensure that the practices were inclusive of all children. For example, for those who found hitting a moving cricket ball challenging, we provided a big tee on which they could place the ball before trying to hit it; once they gained confidence and developed their hand–eye coordination they progressed to a slow-moving ball, and then finally a quicker-moving ball.

Some people in the PE profession didn't like it – they thought it too simplistic (tips for teachers) – but the children and teachers loved it. Many primary-school teachers just aren't into PE and sport; they are classroom teachers who have very limited time during their training on PE (as little as four hours in some cases) so they lack confidence in the wide-open space of the playground. They were glad to have something with structure and content that was as straight-forward as possible.

The next challenge was how to provide the training for 18,000 primary schools on the back of a very small central team. Back then, most local authorities had PE advisors, and we travelled the country persuading them to run the train-ing programmes in their own area. We provided national training and then they cascaded the training to teachers. Every teacher who attended the training got a bag of equip-ment and a set of cards, but not all of them turned up ready to learn. Some would be wearing smart shoes and have handbags over their shoulders, their arms folded as if to say, 'I really don't want to be here, but my headmistress sent me.' But almost all of them became captivated by the ease and accessibility of the activity, joined in readily and ended up having a lot of fun. They enjoyed whacking a ball off a giant tee as much as one of their children.

Within three years, every primary school in the country had a bag of equipment and a set of cards (you can still go into primary schools today and see big blue bags with TOP written on them). However, if I have made it sound like plain sailing, it wasn't! We worked very hard to make it happen and had to raise money constantly to fund the various programmes. Sometimes support came from very unexpected places. One day I happened to meet someone from Ecclesiastical Insurance, which insures Church of England buildings. Following a long conversation about the importance of values, respect and growing young people as role models and leaders, I was invited to speak to their funding committee. They became great partners for our TOP Link programme for a number of years.

In 1994, John Major's Conservative Government introduced specialist schools in England, starting with technology schools and closely followed by language schools. While these schools were expected to be centres of excellence for their chosen specialities, they still taught all the other subjects, and it was hoped that those specialised subjects would drive improvement across the board.

Since starting the YST in 1995, I'd been making a real nuisance of myself at the Department for Education, constantly going into their offices and asking why they weren't spending more money on PE and advocating its importance in school culture and life beyond the school gates. I could clear most of the department in about thirty seconds, and any poor person who hadn't seen me coming would pretend to be on the phone. I had many fruitless conversations, but that didn't stop me speaking to whoever would listen.

The Specialist Schools Trust managed all the specialist colleges (schools), but when John Major wanted some specialist sports colleges they were not eager to take those on as they did not believe they would have a positive impact on overall school standards. Out of the blue I received a call from the Department for Education who invited me to discuss the possibility of the YST taking responsibility for these secondary schools with a sport specialism.

We were offered a small contract and I accepted without fully grasping what we were being asked to do! This was an opportunity to build a relationship with the department and perhaps get some more interest in PE and school sport. I immediately rang Steve Grainger to tell him we had a government contract. It was quite scary, but incredibly exciting.

There was a formal application process and we provided guidance and support for all applicants. In the end eleven schools, rather than ten, were identified, most of whose head teachers had previously taught PE, meaning they could see better than others how sport could improve school stand-ards. Some of them were heads of schools in poor areas, such as Neville Beischer, from Wright Robinson in Gorton, Manchester, where the majority of pupils were eligible for free school meals.

At our first meeting with all eleven heads (we called them our '1st XI'), I started out by explaining that the aim wasn't just for their schools to get better sport, but it was also to use sport as a vehicle to raise academic and behavioural standards. I remember Neville saying, 'How do we do that?' and me replying, 'Well, that's where you come in, because we are going to have to work that out together.'

We started to work out how to make the values in PE and sport – health and well-being, social interaction, inclusivity, fairness, teamwork, discipline, respect and more – the values of the whole school. We were an incredibly tight team, and those head teachers were full of brilliant ideas. Having piloted our plan with our 1st XI, we grew rapidly and had sixty-three sports colleges by 1997.

I'd been told that if Labour won the 1997 election, they might wipe out specialist schools, which would have meant a lot of hard work lost. One of Tony Blair's campaigning slogans was 'education, education, education', and he also happened to be very keen on sport. And when he became Prime Minister, I found his ministers easy to deal with.

Because I worked very closely with the Labour Government, some people assumed I was affiliated with the party. In truth, I am not really a politically motivated person. I do believe that a government should be for everyone, making sure the right things are in place to keep people physically and mentally well. Good health is the basis of a happy, productive society and a strong economy.

The politicians I enjoyed working with most are conviction politicians, who aren't in the job for status, or as a hobby, but who really want to change the world for the better. And Tony Blair's cabinet contained plenty of people like that. They certainly didn't get everything right – no one ever does!

One such person was Estelle Morris, who was Minister for Schools before replacing David Blunkett as Education Secretary in 2001. Like others in Tony Blair's early cabinets – John Prescott, Mo Mowlam, John Reid, Richard Caborn, Tessa Jowell – Estelle had experienced life outside politics. Having attended Whalley Range High School (she was in her final year when I joined), she went on to be a PE and humanities teacher at an inner-city school in Coventry for eighteen years. She understood exactly what education was meant to be about: not just exam results, but giving children the foundations for a good, productive life.

When she was still Minister for Schools, Estelle asked me to help the government develop a strategy for PE and school sport. Coincidentally, Kate Hoey, Minister for Sport, had asked me to do the same thing two days earlier, so I arranged to meet them together. I told them I'd only do it if it was made clear that I was a non-political advisor for both departments – the Department for Education and the Department for Culture, Media and Sport – working in tandem. They readily agreed, and I started planning how to develop a strategy across three government departments: education, health and sport.

Around this time, David Blunkett, who I enjoyed working with, called me in and asked why the sports colleges were improving faster academically than other schools. I explained that the head teachers were using the specialism (sport) to drive a different culture across the school. Then came my first meeting with the PM.

My first impressions of Tony Blair were positive. He had massive charisma; you could feel it whenever he walked into a room. He was easy to talk to and passionate about education and the power of sport to affect change in schools – all music to my ears!

He asked how we could get more schools benefiting from the work of the sports colleges. This was something Steve and I had been working on over our usual beer and crisps on the many train journeys we took together. We agreed we needed a hub-and-spoke model: each sports college to sit at the centre of a family of secondary and primary schools with an infrastructure of people to make it all work.

'How big is each family?' asked the PM.

'That will be dependent on the locality – rural, urban – so each family will need to be designed individually,' I replied.

'How much money do you need?'

'We have estimated that if we pilot this across thirty families it would cost three million pounds to get it off the ground.'

'OK, get it off the ground.'

Now all we had to do was find thirty 'willing' volunteers to take on this challenge and work with them to find out how to take a beacon and spread its light and good practice as far as possible. One thing was for certain: this would not happen without an infrastructure of people. We proposed that each sports college should appoint a full-time partnership development manager, to lead the coordination and cooperation of the schools in the family. We should also invest in a part-time school sport coordinator in each of the six to eight secondary schools (the majority of who were existing PE teachers within the school); and we invited primary schools to put forward a primary link teacher to attend twelve in-service days a year to lead the development of PE across their school. Government money would go direct to the sports colleges, but the YST (the system coach) would also get money for the training and development of everyone in the network.

The PE, School Sport and Club Links strategy, as it was rather inelegantly called, was launched in October 2002. The hub-and-spoke pilot proved so successful that the PM wanted us to roll it out to every school in the country. When he called me in to present at Number 10, it was supposed to be a small meeting. But the pilot scheme had been so successful everyone wanted to hear about it. I ended up presenting to the PM, Culture, Media and Sport Secretary Tessa Jowell, and Charles Clarke – and all their officials, which meant the cabinet room was full to the brim.

We had calculated that we would need more than four hundred sports colleges for every school in the country to be involved in what were now being called School Sport

Partnerships. That's a lot of sports colleges, and a lot of money, which is why I didn't show the slide illustrating roughly how much we would need, but nothing got past Tony Blair. After I finished my presentation, he gave me one of his trademark grins and said, 'I don't suppose you've got the numbers to hand?' I pressed a key on my laptop and the slide revealed that we'd need something like £120 million a year. The PM thought for a moment, then turned to Charles Clarke and said, 'Let's find it.' That was the end of the meeting.

While £120 million sounds like an enormous amount of money, in government terms it's a drop in the ocean. At the time, it was estimated that the NHS cost almost two hundred million pounds a day to run (that figure is now significantly higher), and we were convinced that getting more young people physically active would bring the figure down.

The School Sport Partnerships were a huge success by any measure, and much of the credit must go to the schools and the incredibly dedicated partnership development managers, who worked tirelessly to implement real change across their families of schools.

By 2008, every school (primary, secondary and special) in the country was part of a School Sport Partnership (there were four hundred and fifty in all) and schools had gone from two or three links to sports clubs to twelve or fifteen. In addition, 92 per cent of pupils were doing two hours of sport and PE a week, up from less than 23 per cent in 2002; and over 50 per cent were doing five hours a week. Thousands of young people were doing leadership courses, starting on their journey to becoming future coaches and referees; head teachers were reporting academic and behavioural improvement; and parental engagement had gone up in many schools.

Wright Robinson College, which had been one bad inspection away from being taken over, was voted best school in the country for sport by *The Times* in 2007. The same year, Manchester City Council called it the 'single most improved school or college in the United Kingdom'. Wright Robinson took part in a ten-year research project, in conjunction with the Manchester Institute of Sport and Physical Activity and the YST, which showed that participation in sport and PE significantly improved physical competence, confidence and self-esteem. In addition, 62 per cent of physically active students achieved five or more A$\star$–C GCSEs compared to 38 per cent of the least active.

Looking back, we owe John Major an enormous amount of gratitude for identifying sport as a good cause for Lottery money and greenlighting specialist sports colleges in the first place. He shifted the dial. However, I'm not sure the Conservatives would have moved the sports agenda forward as fast and as far as Tony Blair's government did. While John Major understood the power of sport, I don't think his party did.

In 2007, Tony spoke at a YST conference in Telford. By that time, his star had waned – not only had he taken Britain into protracted wars in Afghanistan and Iraq, but he was also mired in the so-called cash-for-honours scandal, which involved the awarding of life peerages to Labour Party donors. He had been interviewed by the police a few days before the conference, and when he arrived, journalists kept asking what he had told them and when he was going to resign. He ignored all the negativity and was all smiles and chatter with the children who greeted him.

When we finally reached the sanctuary of the green room, he yanked his tie down, his smile disappeared, and suddenly I could see the massive fatigue across his face. He must have had about twenty people with him, but the atmosphere was funereal, with no one saying a word. Finally, I said to him, 'Can I get you a cup of tea?' 'Yes please,' he replied, and we got down to discussing his speech.

He had a speech prepared, but I asked if he could do an extra ten to fifteen minutes at the end, on why sport is such an important part of a child's education. He was only too happy to do that, and when the time came for his speech, he did up his tie, his smile returned, and he was ready for action.

We walked onto the stage together and I said, 'Ladies and gentlemen, I'm not going to introduce our guest to you, because I think you already know him. But, Sir, I would like to introduce the audience to you. This is a can-do audience, full of people who want to change the world. And they want to change it through education and sport.' As he walked to the podium he said jokingly, 'Could you introduce me everywhere I go?'

The prepared speech was all about the impact that these schools were making and the incredible work the network had achieved. The fifteen minutes he ad-libbed at the end were priceless. Despite all the bad stuff that was going on, he was still able to talk with passion and authenticity about the role of sport.

Listening to him, you could tell that his faith in sport to shape character, improve physical and mental health and social well-being came from his heart and his head — it was authentic. And he was very aware that sport at the élite level could inspire people, unite a country, and improve its overall mood (hence why he'd backed London for the 2012 Olympics).

When he was finished, two thousand people stood and applauded. And after we'd left the stage, I noticed that his eyes were moist. He'd entered the venue to journalists asking when he was going to resign, and he'd walked off stage to people clapping and cheering and wanting to shake his hand. That must have been so uplifting for him, a reminder of the good times. I've still got the handwritten note he sent me afterwards: 'On a difficult day, you made me feel very special.'

8

Building a winning team

*Know your own capabilities and surround yourself with people
who shine in those areas which are not your strengths*

Estelle Morris – with whom I worked for four years when I
was CEO of the Youth Sport Trust – was many a head teacher's favourite Education Secretary. She was a woman with
strong values and unwavering principles.

One day, her office called and asked me to come in as
soon as possible. When I walked in, everyone seemed very
upset. And when I asked what was going on, I was told that
Estelle had just resigned as a matter of principle. The PM did
not want her to go, and neither did I, but it was all to no
avail. I found Estelle in her office, distraught. We didn't say
much, but I completely understood the pressure she felt she
was under and the pain of resigning from a job she loved.

Estelle's office let me know when she was going to be
leaving the building for the last time and I made my way to
the Department of Education post-haste. Sanctuary Buildings

in Westminster had a central atrium, overlooked by balconies. And when Estelle appeared in the lobby, ready to make her exit, people on every floor started banging on the glass sides of the atrium. It was such an emotional scene and it melted me. Those civil servants were desperate to show her how special she was (something you certainly wouldn't see nowadays).

One year, I got Estelle to do the closing speech at the YST conference. She was driving up from London to Nottingham, and when the time came for her to appear on stage, she was stuck in traffic. I'd closed all the workshops down, corralled everyone into the main hall and was now standing in front of five hundred head teachers, wittering on about whatever popped into my head. Mercifully, Estelle bounded onto the stage after about twenty minutes, to a huge round of applause. I think they were relieved to be getting rid me!

Estelle told me I didn't need to bother with an introduction, but I wasn't having that. She was getting one whether she liked it or not, because she was such a special person. Once I was done, Estelle delivered a wonderful speech without any notes. She'd been immersed in education for so long, everything she wanted to say was committed to memory. What does it say about politics, I thought, that somebody so knowledgeable, genuine, and committed could not survive its brutality.

The success of the school sport programme meant that I had gained a reputation for solving challenges. So after the 2000

Olympics and Paralympics in Sydney, I was asked to support veteran MP Jack Cunningham with a report into the funding of élite sport in the UK. The Cunningham report was published in 2002, and the recommendations laid the foundation for my future role as chair of UK Sport.

The following year, I went to meet Tessa Jowell to report on the progress of the school sport programme. She was still in a sports cabinet meeting, with the ministers for Scotland, Wales and Northern Ireland, the CEOs of Sport England, Sport Scotland, Sport Wales and Sport Northern Ireland (as the Sports Councils had become), and the chair and chief executive of UK Sport. I've no idea what went on in that meeting, but when she returned to her office, she was not amused. Tessa wasn't one to shout and scream and throw things around, but she was as close to being angry as I'd ever seen her.

I suggested to her private secretary Helen MacNamara that we reschedule, but Tessa insisted that our meeting go ahead.

Tessa proceeded to tell me what had gone on in the meeting, and that she had come to the conclusion that élite sport in the UK needed reforming. The British Olympic Association had been working on a bid to host the 2012 Olympics since 1997, the year Labour came to power, and I think Tessa wanted to be able to say to Tony Blair with confidence, 'If we host the Olympics, we'll be more successful than ever.' Then she came out with it:

'Would you like to do it?'

'Do what?' I replied, somewhat startled.

'Be the reform chair of UK Sport.'

'I've come to talk to you about school sport! And I've never chaired anything in my life.'

'Don't worry about that. I need you to go in and reform it.'

'What needs doing?'

'Find out if UK Sport is doing what it should. And if we even need it.'

I was CEO of the YST, so I had to ask Sir John Beckwith, who paid my wages, if he'd be OK with me doing two days a week at UK Sport. 'If it's going to make British sport better,' he replied, 'go for it.' That was typical Sir John, although if he'd known how much time I'd actually spend at UK Sport over the coming years, he might not have agreed so readily.

My job as reform chair was to look at the system and work out if and how it could be improved, or whether UK Sport should merge with Sport England. As is my wont, I spent the first few weeks listening and asking lots of questions, just to get a feel for the place. People weren't used to the chair wandering about the building, let alone making lots of cups of tea in the kitchen, and I'd listen in on all their gossiping. I also went round the office, sitting next to each colleague at their desk and asking three simple questions: 'What do you do? What could you do? What stops you?' They may sound like simple questions, but the answers are very revealing.

I had three buckets of people in my head: bucket one: creative people, who thought and did things differently and conjured new ideas; bucket two: 'engine people', who weren't going to come up with new ideas but were going to work hard, focus on the mission and drive the changes I wanted to see; and bucket three: people who needed to work somewhere else. The answers to the questions revealed many things about the quality of the individuals and the management style which was predominantly 'tell' rather than 'empower and unlock creativity'.

One of our roles as leaders of organisations, just like the coach of a team, is to understand the talents and limitations of every individual so that we can help each of them fulfil their potential. Growing your people is the key to great organisations. It is important to take the time to find out who your people are and what they know, before moving them around to play to their strengths: if you put them in a box and never let them out again, they'll slowly wither. Talent is often hidden and needs nurturing. Managing people is a bit like gardening: you have to buy (recruit) plants (people) that can thrive in the area of the garden (business) you want them to work in. You need to prepare the soil well (great induction), ensure you water regularly (feedback) and put the plant in the sunlight (let them shine).

I soon realised that the mindset needed improving across the board, because there were too many people working there who thought British sport was doing just fine. One day, I asked some of my new colleagues if they thought finishing tenth in the medal table, which Team GB had done at the 2000 Olympics in Sydney, was a good result. Someone replied, 'Well, it's better than thirty-sixth,' referring to the 1996 Olympics in Atlanta, where we'd won only one gold medal.

'That wasn't my question,' I said. 'Do you think tenth is good?'

No one spoke. Eventually I said, 'I've never wanted to be tenth in my life. Why would anybody be satisfied with tenth?'

I started going through all the countries that finished above us in Sydney and asking why they were better than us, and my colleagues kept telling me it was because their athletes had better talent systems, more insight data on world standards, better sports science and sports medicine, greater innovation and so on. To which I responded, 'But why are they better at these things than us, and how do we change the way we do things to take us to a new level?'

There was a lot of talk about being world-class at UK Sport, but that had to begin with us. We had to model the best, not simply talk about it. Everything: from the way we greeted people at reception, to how we dealt with our partners, the standards we set in meetings and how we modelled openness and transparency with the media. It is not possible to drive excellence unless you are walking the walk.

After a couple of months, I went back to see Tessa Jowell and told her I believed we could transform UK Sport into the high-performance organisation she wanted but that there needed to be some fundamental changes and I would need her backing. 'What are you going to do, dear?' she said, and I replied, 'First of all, I have to change the majority of the senior team, including the chief executive.' Her eyes widened. 'We need to be world-class, agile, innovative and cutting edge if we are to transform the culture and take us to the next level.' To do that we needed fresh minds and a fresh approach.

I decided that Richard Callicott (CEO) was not the right person to lead this change agenda. Richard had been in the role for four years, and while he was a good man and popular with the staff I simply didn't believe he was the right fit at this time. Not that telling him was easy.

We were at a meeting with the Sports Council for Wales in Cardiff when I decided it was time. I asked him to join me for a walk along the river, and I think he could sense something was coming. 'Richard,' I said, 'you're a good man, but we need very different leadership if we are going to drive the system forward.' Understandably, he was upset and I hoped he wouldn't get angry in case he was tempted to push me into the river!

Most people are trying their best, which is why telling people that they're no longer needed is the hardest thing you ever have to do. If anybody ever tells you it's easy and just part of a boss's job, they're not normal. Even to this day it keeps me up all night beforehand, and the aftermath is horrible. Self-respect is the most precious possession of any individual.

UK Sport's head of anti-doping, Michele Verroken, also moved on, which was not without controversy. Over time everyone at senior management level left except for John Scott in International development and Liz Nicholl, a former Wales netball international whom I had coached at university. Liz, who had done great things as chief executive of the All England Netball Association and joined UK Sport as director of élite sport in 1999, was very highly respected by all the NGBs of sport.

Following a series of interviews, I appointed John Steele as the new CEO in 2005. John had left the army to pursue a career as a professional rugby player and was a very successful fly-half for Northampton. He was a charismatic leader and had a clear understanding of sporting excellence. He left UK Sport to take up his dream job as CEO of the Rugby Football Union (RFU) in 2010. John immediately conducted a comprehensive review at the RFU, but this led to considerable turbulence and he departed after nine months in the post.

My new head of communications was Tim Hollingsworth, who had not worked in sport before. He was an outstanding appointment and after leaving UK Sport he became the CEO of the British Paralympic Association and led the organisation into four Paralympic Games before becoming the Chief Executive of Sport England in 2018.

Now all I needed to complete the team was a new performance director: someone who would bring experience and blue-sky thinking to the party.

I first met Peter Keen when I awarded him a prize for being the outstanding sports science student of the year. Peter did a sports studies degree at University College

Chichester before completing a Master of philosophy degree in exercise physiology at Loughborough University. Then in 1992, Pete, who had been a talented cyclist in his youth, coached Chris Boardman to Britain's first Olympic gold medal in cycling for seventy-two years. Pete had played a big part in the aforementioned Cunningham report, and throughout our meetings he impressed me with his insights and clarity of thought – he had an extraordinary mind.

Having become British Cycling's performance director in 1997, Pete transformed Britain into a cycling powerhouse. At the 2004 Olympics in Athens, Britain finished third in the cycling medal table with two golds (Bradley Wiggins and Chris Hoy), while at the 2004 Paralympics, Britain finished fourth in the medal table with three golds.

By the time I arrived at UK Sport, Pete had joined pharmaceutical and biotechnology giant GlaxoSmithKline as performance director of its science sports academy (Dave Brailsford replaced him as British Cycling's performance director before the 2004 Olympics), but I wondered if he could be tempted to join me at UK Sport and mastermind our medal-winning strategy.

I tracked Pete down and asked him to meet me for dinner. During our meal I said, 'I have a dream.' Pete looked at me quizzically. 'I believe we can be the most successful Olympic and Paralympic nation in the world for our population size.' I paused for a moment. 'But I can't do it without you.'

Pete gave it some thought, then said, 'I can't do that. I'm married, I've got a small child. And I'm earning good money.'

'Oh. OK. Can you give me any time at all?'

'I don't think so, no.'

That was something of an anticlimax, and I thought I'd have to look elsewhere. But Pete phoned me a couple of weeks later and asked if he could do the role in a part-time capacity. 'I'll take whatever you can give me,' I said, 'we just need your brain.'

Having put me in touch with his bosses, Pete then went quiet again. When he finally called and said he wanted to meet me, I thought he was going to tell me he'd had a change of heart. I started off by telling him I respected him whatever decision he had made, and that I knew I'd put him in a difficult situation, and he said, 'I share your dream and I'd like to work with you.' He left GlaxoSmithKline altogether, and joined us, completing the new dream team of John, Tim, Liz and Pete – the journey could begin!

Disrupting an entire sporting system did not come without its challenges. There was a well-established way of doing things but that needed to radically change. We needed to begin by sharing a vision of what was possible and take the home country sports council and the NGBs with us on the journey. The first step was to disrupt our way of thinking internally. There were plenty of heated discussions and differences of opinion, but we kept coming back to 'What will make this system go faster and further?'

A number of politicians thought we needed one big institute of sport in the middle of the country, like they had in

Australia (having won no gold medals at the 1976 Olympics, which was regarded as a national embarrassment, Australia opened their Institute of Sport in Canberra in 1981 and were among the most successful sporting nations in the world by the 1990s).

The Australian concept of a central sports institute was brilliant: put your best athletes with the best coaches and best sports scientists all under one roof, with the best facilities. It sounds so simple, but I wondered if that would necessarily work in the UK. For a start, the UK is made up of four different countries. Second, we already had great infrastructures in established clubs. So we could learn from the concept and practice of the Australian model, but adapt it to our unique sporting infrastructure. So there was one centralised venue for cycling – the velodrome in Manchester – but in other sports we needed two or three different high-performance centres to accommodate our athletes.

Of course, there is always much to learn from other countries, but the trick is to adapt elements of different systems for your existing culture, rather than picking them up and trying to hammer them in, like square pegs into round holes.

When I first joined UK Sport, I began by asking questions. One of the first questions I asked was how funding was allocated and why. I was told that each governing body wrote a plan and UK Sport gave them money depending on the quality of the plan. So, I asked them to give me six random plans, without telling me how much money each sport had received, and I took them home and studied them over the weekend, paying particular attention to how many major medals each sport had won in recent years. In other words, was the plan working and were we getting anything back for the money we were investing?

Of the six plans, the gymnastics plan was good, but the results did not match the ambition. When I returned to work on Monday and asked how much money gymnastics was getting, I was told that it received more than the other five sports.

I said, 'What am I missing?'

'What do you mean?'

'Why are we giving gymnastics that much money?'

'Because they wrote a really good plan.'

'We're not giving out Pulitzer Prizes. Where are the medals?'

'Beth Tweddle is World and European champion—'

'That's one gymnast. And we haven't won a gymnastics medal at the Olympics since 1928. Where's the pathway? Where are the young performers coming through?'

They tried to argue, but you cannot give money out based on a persuasive plan, hoping that somewhere along the road it will turn into gold. This was public money, given to us by the government and the Lottery, so we needed to start spending it more responsibly, rather than frittering it away on pipe dreams.

I reflected on a conversation I had with my dad when I was a child. Every Saturday night, he'd take me with him to the shops and have me count up the tills and bag the money.

This was all designed to help me with my arithmetic, which was not one of my strong points. One day, I said to Dad, 'We've made a lot of money today, how are you going to spend it?' And he replied, 'The taxman will take a good chunk of it.'

'Who is this taxman?'

'The government.'

'Why do they take our money?'

'That's just how it works.'

'What do they do with it?'

'It goes to fund things like schools and hospitals. I only hope they use it wisely.'

At UK Sport, we were spending taxpayers' money, so I wanted us to be as wise with it as if we were investing our own money. We were investing money in the sports, so we needed to see a return. If we didn't, we would have to think about putting our money elsewhere, which was going to make some people angry. Most of all, we needed to be cleverer, which is where the amazing Peter Keen comes in.

Pete sharing my dream was one thing, but he could also visualise what a successful system needed to look like in granular detail. At that point, the four home nations' sports councils funded their talented podium potential athletes (eight years from the podium) and UK Sport only got involved in the last four years (podium athletes). Pete was adamant that we needed to be involved in the last eight years if we wanted to effect long-term change. That meant taking responsibility – and in some cases money – from the home country sports councils, which was difficult to explain and even harder to deliver. But with patience, political backing and a lot of perseverance we succeeded.

We also needed more accountability, because there were too many sports handing in grand plans, delivering another set of average results and then making excuses. To that end, Pete came up with the idea of investing in individual athletes.

Pete spent untold hours working out a cost analysis per athlete, using data from the most successful countries in the world. Essentially, he calculated roughly how many hours of work (coaching, analysis, nutrition, psychology, etc.) needed to go into an athlete to make them successful on the world stage.

We then said to the various performance directors, 'Name me the athletes who are going to win medals in major championships in the next four years. And the potential winners in the four years after that.' They also had to show us why they thought those athletes were going to win medals. On that basis we then allocated the funding based on the number of athletes and asked them to write the plan based on those individuals – an athlete-centred approach to funding.

When I introduced the phrase 'no compromise', some in the media misinterpreted it. The interpretation was that we wanted sports to be ultra-hard on athletes, a throwback to the sporting regimes in Eastern Europe. What we actually meant was that if we wanted our athletes to achieve their best possible results, we couldn't compromise on any element of their support and preparation. To be the best you have to be surrounded by the best.

If someone has the talent and ambition and is prepared to put in the work and make the necessary sacrifices to be the best in the world, I don't want to let them down. I don't want them to look at me after an Olympics and say, 'If only you'd given me a better coach, if only you'd given me a better psychologist, if only you'd given me a better nutritionist, if only you'd given me more warm-weather training . . .'

Our job at UK Sport was to eliminate the 'if onlys', because that's the only way to give your athletes a fair chance of succeeding on the world stage. Olympic and Paralympic athletes sacrifice a huge amount – social life, family life, earning potential – for not much financial reward. Unlike élite male footballers, they don't retire with a big house and a garage full of sports cars. But they might retire with a gold medal and the satisfaction that they fulfilled their dream. And if I could help them achieve that, I didn't see it as being ruthless or unscrupulous. I saw it as my moral duty.

We were also accused of giving too much money to so-called posh sports, such as rowing, sailing and equestrian, at the expense of sports that were more accessible to a less privileged, and more diverse, demographic. But while I'd always believed in the inspirational power of sport – and understood the argument that it didn't matter how many sailing medals we won, it was unlikely to inspire someone who didn't live near water or have the money to sail a boat – I was also acutely aware that, as chair of UK Sport, my purpose was to invest in potential success and win as many medals as possible. What value can be placed on national pride and the power of the role models we generate who, through their own endeavour, achieve their dreams?

That meant that some sports, like basketball and volley-ball, did not get investment because at that time they were not within reach of success on the Olympic or Paralympic stage. They needed investment from the home country sports councils to grow participation, develop a talent pathway and develop more coaches and officials. When you consider a range of investment propositions you must select those that will give the greatest return. It was the same principle for winter sports, but where we did have real prospects, such as skeleton and bobsleigh, we invested accordingly.

The mindset had changed: it was no longer about just taking part and backing as many athletes as possible, it was about backing those who had a chance of making the podium. We invested heavily in athletics, swimming and boxing, three sports with global reach that meant they faced even greater challenges to bring home medals.

The CEO of British Gymnastics was Alan Sommerville, who I'd met when I was working in the East Midlands. And when I brought him in for a meeting and told him that we were drastically reducing his budget, he looked at me in horror and said, 'You can't do that.' 'I know this is tough, but we need to focus on gymnasts now and in the future that can achieve world-class standards,' I replied.

I explained that we would give Beth Tweddle, who was Britain's first female gymnast to win European and World Championship medals, all the support she needed – the best coaches, the best facilities, the best sports science and a cohort of training partners – to give her the best possible chance of success, but Alan was still unhappy.

'But, Alan, you haven't got any other medal hopefuls,' I said.

'We'll never have any others now,' he replied.

In the end, I said, 'Tell you what, you go away and identify a group of gymnasts who are about six to eight years away from being medal prospects but have proven ability at their age group, and we will invest in them.' Alan still wasn't happy, but that was my final offer. Alan decided on a group of young male gymnasts who were winning plenty of junior medals in artistic gymnastics.

I'll never forget him saying to me, 'When we win a medal in London, I'm going to find you and say, "Now give me your money!"' I replied: 'If you win a medal in London, Alan, that will be the start of a very different conversation.'

I earned a reputation for making tough decisions in the pursuit of success, but I'm not sure that there's any other way to become world-leading.

We brought in people to challenge the way we were thinking, we took external advice on every piece of proposed reform, we brought in government experts to look at our proposed governance changes, and we always consulted with the home nations' sports councils. I was like a mechanic, meticulously dismantling a machine and seeing if it could be put back together in a different, more effective way.

My view was that UK Sport and the four home nations' sports councils needed to work in partnership, with a combined mission to produce the best high-performance system in the world. I felt UK Sport should provide mission leadership, but that is not how things had operated in the past and would require our relationships to be reset.

It became confrontational and at times was excruciatingly uncomfortable. I often felt that the challenges were personal and struggled to deal with the anguish it caused. But change was needed and I remained resolved to face into the storm.

Leadership is about remaining positive and dealing with the pain privately. Resilience comes from being clear about the mission – the job to be done – and not allowing personal attacks to drive you off course.

It was a political power struggle. I was this person who wanted to make changes that were going to disrupt the existing system and – in their view – reduce their influence.

What they hadn't grasped was that I wasn't interested in power. All I was interested in was completing my mission, which was to make Great Britain the most successful Olympic and Paralympic nation in the world for its popula-tion size. And while I couldn't know for sure if my changes would work as planned, I did know that if we carried on doing what we'd always done, we'd get what we'd always got.

The evening before the sports cabinet meeting where my reform papers were due to go in, I was grilled for an hour by the chairs of the home nations' sports councils. Their gist was that my proposed changes had no hope of being accepted and the meeting was going to be a disaster. They even suggested I pull the papers to save myself from humiliation. When they'd finished making their points, I said to them, 'It's very interesting that we've talked for an hour and none of you has mentioned our joint ambition to become the most successful Olympic and Paralympic nation. But, I hear you. You don't like what I'm doing, and that's your prerogative. Are we done?' If that makes me sound steely, that's not how I was feeling on the inside. It was a horrible experience. And when I got back to my room, the strain and emotion hit me hard.

Suddenly the phone rang. It was Richard Caborn, Minister for Sport, and he was his usual chirpy self. 'What's the matter with you?' he said in his thick Yorkshire accent, and while I was trying to explain, he said, 'Get down here now. You need a whisky.' 'I don't drink whisky,' I said. 'You do tonight!' he replied.

When I walked into the hotel lounge at about eleven o'clock, he slammed a bottle of whisky on the desk, poured me a glass and I forced it down. When I explained what the chairs had said to me, Richard responded, 'They're forgetting one thing, love – I am the chuffin' Minister for Sport! Leave it to me . . .'

I wasn't confident that Richard would be able to do anything because the meeting was at ten the following morning. But as it turned out, all my reforms went through without a hitch. I spent the whole meeting looking at the sports council chairs, waiting for the revolt, but it never came. In fact, they barely looked up from their desks, let alone tried to start a revolution.

Richard has never told me what went on. Maybe he spoke directly to the chairs, maybe he spoke to the ministers for Scotland, Wales and Northern Ireland and asked them to tell their respective chairs that resistance was futile. Whatever took place, they were still angry with me afterwards, two of them in particular. They didn't shout and scream, but they let me know that I'd get my comeuppance eventually. But it didn't really matter what they thought any more, because UK Sport now officially had authority to modernise and move forward.

There is a Nike video I love titled 'Rise and Shine'. It shows various athletes training and competing, including a runner slipping and sliding down the side of a mountain, accompanied by a motivational narration. Here's the part that I really relate to:

'For what is each day but a series of conflicts between the right way and the easy way?'

The video goes on to compare the easy way to several streams heading downhill, and the right way to heading upstream. In heading upstream, you actively 'decide to turn your back on what's comfortable and safe'. You choose the hard option, against other people's advice, because the end result is just that important. After all, as the video puts it, 'the easy way out will always be there, ready to wash you away . . .'

Trying to change the status quo and make the world a better place is never easy, and I often say to people, 'If you want to be at the cutting edge, expect to get cut.' It's not that I see myself as some heroic crusader, flying into battle with no concern for my own well-being, but my passion is so deep that I have to choose the right way, rather than the way that is *comfortable and safe and what some would call common sense*. That's my definition of integrity.

9

Doing what is right

*Integrity is having the courage to do what is
right, not what is popular or expedient*

I was confirmed as permanent chair of UK Sport in 2005,
which meant Steve Grainger becoming CEO and me
becoming Chair of the Youth Sport Trust. It was a heavy
workload, but I enjoyed it immensely because it felt like I
was making a difference.

In the background, the bidding process for the 2012
Olympics was inching forward. In May 2004, the International Olympic Committee (IOC) whittled the candidates down to five cities, with Paris the red-hot favourite
and London considered a long shot. Even after Seb Coe
took over as chairman of the London bid, it took a while for
us to get our messaging right.

At one of our presentations to the IOC's selection committee, our delegation consisted of ten white men in suits and
ties, Tessa Jowell and me, stuck on the end of the row. When

Seb started talking about London being one of the most multi-cultural cities in the world, it didn't look like it.

Afterwards, I said to Seb, 'Great speech. But do you know what we've just done?'

'What?' said Seb.

'One of the most multi-cultural cities in the world? Look at us!'

That started a discussion about how we might do things differently when we travelled to Singapore for the final vote in July 2005. Every city was going to say that their stadium was the best (Paris's was already built and had been the centrepiece of a World Cup seven years earlier), and that they had the best facilities, the best transport system. The others in the running would all be able to promise better weather than London . . . or so we thought. So instead of taking one hundred adult delegates to Singapore like everyone else, we decided to take seventy adults and thirty young people from a specialist sports college in East London who were representative of the community that would be most affected by the London Games.

For two days, Tony Blair and his wife Cherie received IOC members in their hotel suite and tried to persuade them of the virtues of a London Olympics. Seb, who knows all about the importance of preparation, was part of a small team who spent four or five days on the island of Sentosa, fine-tuning the final presentation, including his all-important closing remarks.

David Beckham was also there, and there were few bigger sports stars in the world at the time. Crucially, he didn't just come along as a mascot; he attended all the receptions, visited schools, played football with the pupils and presented prizes. Some people had a negative view of David because of how he was portrayed in the media, but I found him completely unaffected by his enormous fame. He was polite and approachable, a patriotic, passionate ambassador, who really wanted to help.

When we turned up to the Raffles City Convention Centre on election day – 6 July 2005 – things looked very different. The auditorium was a sea of men in suits, except for our secret weapons – thirty very excited young people.

The day began with each city's final forty-five-minute pitch, Paris going first and London fourth. Paris's pitch predictably focused on venues, transport systems and regeneration strategies, and their main film, which was created by famous movie director Luc Besson, looked like a tourism advert. In contrast, London's pitch was about inspiring children all over the world to play sport.

Seb spoke about the need for the Olympic movement to connect to young people, to safeguard the Games themselves. He described how, as a boy at school, he'd watched – on a black-and-white TV – John and Sheila Sherwood, a husband-and-wife duo from his home town of Sheffield, win medals at the 1968 Olympics, and how it had inspired him to become an athlete.

'My heroes were Olympians,' he said. 'My children's heroes change by the month. And they are the lucky ones. Millions more face the obstacle of limited resources, and the resulting lack of guiding role models. Today we offer London's vision of inspiration and legacy. Choose London today and you send a clear message to the youth of the world: more than ever, the Olympic Games are for you.' It was stirring stuff.

Our main film, made in just five weeks by Darryl Goodrich and Caroline Rowland, both based in London, was a master-stroke. Instead of sweeping views of London's famous land-marks, which everyone had seen a thousand times before, it showed two boys and two girls watching the 2012 Olympics in London – and being inspired to become athletes them-selves and dreaming of Olympic success.

Deliberately, and crucially, none of the children in the film was British. One boy is sitting in front of a ramshackle shop somewhere in Africa, throwing stones at tin cans, when he hears commentary and turns to see a TV show-ing a Nigerian winning the 100m in London. One girl is sitting in her front room somewhere in China, listening to music on her headphones, when she becomes mesmerised by a Chinese gymnast performing in London. There is also a shy, withdrawn Russian girl watching swimming and a South American boy watching track cycling, while eating a snack. It then shows each child's progress, from tiny beginners to promising teenagers, ending with the African boy, now a man, on the starting blocks in an Olympic 100m final.

After the presentation, there was a feeling that London suddenly had a chance. We led Paris by one vote after the first round, but when Moscow was eliminated, most of their votes shifted to Madrid, who surged ahead after round two. But when New York fell by the wayside, most of their votes swung to London, meaning Madrid was eliminated and it was us and Paris in the final head-to-head.

During the build-up, there had apparently been talk of a mutual support act between London and Madrid, whereby as soon as one city was eliminated, its supporters would switch allegiances to the other. Seb was also friends with Spain's former IOC President Juan Antonio Samaranch, who remained very influential. But Paris had failed with bids for the 1992 and 2008 Games, so we wondered if the IOC might find it difficult to turn them down again.

We had been in the auditorium for hours when IOC President Jacques Rogge took to the stage and requested the envelope containing the name of the winning city. By this point, the thirty East End pupils were climbing up the walls. I must have been asked, 'What do you think, Miss? Are we going to do it?' a thousand times. We also talked about what should happen if we lost – dignified losers then cry later, me included!

Then, as the envelope was being delivered, on a silk pillow by a young navy cadet, I felt two small hands grasp mine on either side. I looked around to see that all the young people had linked hands, which was a beautiful moment.

I'm pretty sure that Jacques Rogge doesn't open his own post because he took forever to open the envelope. Even after he had opened it, it took him ages to tell us who'd won: 'The International Olympic Committee has the honour of announcing that the Games of the 30th Olympiad in 2012 are awarded to the city of L—'

That's all I heard. Next thing I knew, bodies were falling on top of me and all I could hear was people screeching, 'We've done it! We've done it!'

London would host the 2012 Olympic Games, that much was certain. How many medals we would win depended on how much money we could 'persuade' the government to give us. That may sound mercenary, but the reality is that if you want to be among the best in the world, it needs investment. I wonder how people in Britain felt after Team GB won a single gold medal at the 1996 Games in Atlanta?

Pete had meticulously worked out how much money we'd need for Team GB to finish fourth in the medal table in London, which was the height of our ambition. We accepted that the United States and China would finish ahead of us, and probably Russia, but Pete had set a target of sixty-five medals, which we thought would be enough to leapfrog the likes of Australia and Germany.

It was my job to take Pete's calculations to Chancellor of the Exchequer Gordon Brown and request the necessary cash – and Gordon and I had a bit of history.

Back in 2003, I'd negotiated a partnership between the YST and Cadbury, as in the people who make chocolate bars. Our discussions with Cadbury were about creating a programme called Get Active, helping young people begin to understand the balance between energy in and energy out. Whatever fuel you put in the engine you need to balance with activity if you want to stay fit and healthy. Paula Radcliffe helped us launch the campaign, because she was sponsored by Cadbury and ate lots of chocolate – but also ran lots of miles.

Unfortunately, one of the newspapers ran a story claiming that by offering sports kit in exchange for tokens from chocolate bar wrappers, we were exacerbating the country's childhood obesity problem. That was the complete opposite of what we wanted, but I should have been more savvy and realised the media would turn it into a negative story.

Along with the head of Cadbury's marketing team I was summoned to Number 11 Downing Street, where we were harangued by a range of health experts. We pulled the initiative straight away. While we had been misinterpreted, our message hadn't been clear enough. Another hard lesson about the media.

Thankfully, Gordon had put all that behind him. Still, asking for more money when the Olympics was already costing so much was going to be very challenging.

Pete and I presented our business case to the Treasury officials. Pete had done meticulous preparation, and there wasn't one thing in that plan that he couldn't back up with evidence, so any scepticism was soon washed away. We showed how much money we'd need to finish eighth, sixth and fourth in the medal table. We tried to impress on them that it was essentially a credible business plan, not wishful thinking on our part. The bottom line was that to finish fourth, we would need an additional three hundred million pounds between

2006 and 2012, fifty million a year, double what they were already giving us. I left the meeting hopeful that we had persuaded Treasury officials to give our business plan serious consideration.

While I was at the 2006 Commonwealth Games in Melbourne, Seb got a call from Gordon Brown to say that he was only going to give us an extra two hundred million pounds. I explained that this would mean we would only finish eighth in the medal table. And the message came back that he wanted us to finish fourth. 'No,' I said. 'That's only going to happen if we get the extra three hundred million.' We went back and forth for months, until eventually Gordon Brown announced in his March 2007 budget speech that the funding of Britain's élite athletes would be doubled over the next six years to six hundred million, with two hundred million of additional central government funding and one hundred million from private-sector sponsorship.

That was all well and good, but where was this one hundred million going to come from? Time passed, and we had completed the four-year planning cycle for London and wanted to announce the funding allocation for each sport to allow them to appoint or retain key staff and start their journey to the Olympics. To approve the proposed funding, we had a Board meeting in the diary but did still not have the additional one hundred million from the private sector. This meant we could get the main medal sports announced but others would have to wait in the hope the money could be found.

The day before the meeting I was called in to see Andy Burnham, Secretary of State for the Department of Digital, Culture, Media and Sport (DCMS). Andy and I had a good relationship, but I knew this was going to be tough. He wanted me to postpone the meeting so they could have longer to find the additional funding. I explained that we could not keep sports waiting any longer and any delay would jeopardise our chances of achieving the target we had agreed. Andy was adamant, but so was I. So much depended on this moment. The easiest personal decision would have been to have agreed to postpone the Board meeting, but the mission required me to stay firm and resolute – doing what was right, not what was popular or expedient. It was an uncomfortable experience, but when I left I was determined that the Board meeting would proceed.

Then another phone call came from DCMS to let me know that some of the one hundred million (enough for us to move forward) would be made available by the government and we could announce all sports the next day. We now had no excuses: all the sports had a level of funding that would allow them to appoint the best coaches and afford the very latest in sports science, research and development.

To drive further innovation we had a central team whose job was to uncover any piece of technology or science that might give our athletes an advantage, however small – what Dave Brailsford famously referred to as 'marginal gains'. We worked with British Aerospace and the Formula 1 team McLaren, who gave us access to key personnel and technology, such as their air tunnels that allowed us to create more aerodynamic helmets for cyclists. Through our many partnerships we searched out cutting-edge expertise that could enhance our athletes' chances of success on the world stage. Sports themselves began researching and gathering data to inform practice in a way that had not been done before. The performance system was really taking shape and people were embracing the changes.

Some journalists wanted to believe that our success was all down to money, or what some people referred to as 'financial doping', which implied that we were cheating in some way. The reality is that the pursuit of excellence at the highest level is extremely expensive – just look at Formula 1. And just as Formula 1 teams pair their best drivers with their best cars and their best mechanics, we had to do the same: identify the best talent under the guidance of the best coaches and support them with the best sports science and sports medicine. While everyone who competes at the highest level works extremely hard and has talent, not everyone has the self-belief to become a winner. Through the environment we were creating, individuals began to believe they had the best support in the world, so they stepped forward with greater confidence.

Money was important, but our success was much more than that. It was built on great people in the sports themselves. The performance directors in each sport who masterminded the execution of the plans, the brilliant coaches whose dedication and commitment can often be overlooked and that army of sports science and sports medicine experts providing extensive individual and team support. At UK Sport the team did a terrific job lead by Pete Keen, the principal architect, and Liz Nicholl whose constancy, credibility and honesty built the partnerships with sports that made all this possible.

Better never stops, which is why you can never be complacent with your system. High performance stems from restlessness, from people who are never satisfied. That's why the great coaches never think they know all the answers, but instead are always asking, 'What's next?' For example, a few weeks after leading England to the Rugby World Cup in 2003, Clive Woodward came to see me at UK Sport. When he could have been basking in the glory, instead he wanted to know what the next big sports science frontier might be. Clive knew that while his England team had shown themselves to be the best in the world, they could not stand still because other nations are constantly improving.

For many years, British sporting success usually involved a visionary coach just happening to unite with a group of unusually talented athletes at exactly the right time – only to be followed by years of underachievement.

England's men's football team hasn't won a major tournament since the 1966 World Cup, when Alf Ramsey was united with the likes of Bobby Moore, Bobby Charlton and Gordon Banks, all world-class talents. England's men's rugby union team has never reached anything like the same heights since winning the World Cup in 2003, when Clive Woodward was united with the likes of Jonny Wilkinson, Martin Johnson and Jason Robinson.

In Olympic sport, there was that great era of men's middle-distance runners in the early 1980s, led by Seb Coe, Steve Ovett and Steve Cram. But that wasn't a system: that was just three exceptional talents with exceptional coaches who broke through at roughly the same time. After Seb's 1500m gold medal at the 1984 Olympics, a British male didn't win a global title in a middle-distance event until Jake Wightman in the 1500m at the 2022 World Championships.

Then there was the GB men's hockey team that won gold in 1988, when Roger Self and David Whitaker united with the likes of Sean Kerly, Imran Sherwani and Ian Taylor. Roger was an unconventional manager who had revived Great Britain's fortunes after decades of decline, while David was the brilliant head coach he appointed. But because of the system they were working in, sustaining success was difficult.

Of course, you've got to find the right managers and coaches, but they're just part of the puzzle. If the rest of the puzzle is confused, even the greatest managers and coaches will fail. That's why Roger's greatest legacy to the sport was probably the Framework Agreement signed by England, Scotland and Wales in 2006, when he was president of GB Hockey. This prioritised Great Britain's success at the Olympics and paved the way for another revival. With investment support from UK Sport the women's team won bronze at London 2012, gold at Rio 2016 and bronze again at Tokyo 2020.

One of the other big factors in developing any sporting system is the talent pathway. I was particularly interested in why our women weren't winning more medals (Denise Lewis was the only woman to win a medal at the 1996 Olympics in Atlanta, bronze in the heptathlon, and women won about 30 per cent of our medals in 2000 in Sydney). Was it a lack of support, or a lack of female talent?

We had done well in women's rowing, winning a silver medal at the 2000 Olympics and two more in 2004, but we couldn't just say, 'Well, hopefully they'll win us another medal in 2008' – we had to be more proactive and work out how to unearth more women with medal-winning potential.

Chelsea Warr worked at the Australian Institute of Sport before taking a job at British Diving and Swimming. She joined UK Sport in 2005 and pioneered Britain's talent identification programme, which identified and fast-tracked hundreds of athletes. Our most successful talent-spotting initiative was Sporting Giants, which was launched by five-time Olympic rowing champion Sir Steve Redgrave in Trafalgar Square in 2007. About four thousand people applied and they were tested in groups of two hundred, with the experts primarily interested in potential rowers, canoers, volleyballers and handball players.

Candidates had to be tall (a minimum of six feet three inches for men and five feet eleven inches for women), aged between sixteen and twenty-five and have some kind of athletic background (I believe we also asked if their parents had any sporting prowess). And one of the women who applied was Helen Glover, a former junior England hockey player and runner who also represented Cornwall in swimming and tennis.

Helen talks about arriving at the National Sports Centre in Bisham Abbey and someone saying, 'A gold medallist in 2012 could be sat in this room. Look around you.' Helen decided that person would be her.

She'd lied about her height – she was five feet ten inches and stood on tiptoes while being measured – but demonstrated unbelievable heart and lung function. However, identifying Helen's talent was just the first part of the process, because it could only be confirmed once we'd put her on a talent development programme.

Yes, an athlete might look the part, but it's only when you put them on a talent pathway that you discover whether they have all the other attributes that are required to succeed at the highest level, such as work ethic, resilience, mental toughness, and the ability to listen and learn fast. If they do demonstrate all those important traits over a set period of time, you then arrive at the talent confirmation point when you can increase the investment to help them travel all the way to the podium.

As it turned out, Helen did have what it takes, in spades. Having been placed in GB Rowing's Team Start programme, she won a silver at the World Rowing Championships in 2010, alongside Heather Stanning, another talent-programme graduate who had only been rowing for four years. They also produced the first gold medal performance of the London Olympic Games – what a moment!

Sporting Giants identified fifty-eight athletes who were then placed in Olympic development programmes, but it wasn't our only way of identifying talent. Four times as many men as women having applied for Sporting Giants, Girls4Gold was aimed at women between seventeen and twenty-five who had competed at county level or above in any sport. Successful applicants were introduced to either cycling, canoeing, rowing, sailing, modern pentathlon or the winter sport of skeleton. Lizzy Yarnold, a former heptathlete, was identified as a potential medal winner in skeleton, and within two years she was competing and winning on the international circuit. She'd go on to win two gold medals at the 2014 and 2018 Winter Olympics.

Despite what the cynics might have said, I never lost my idealism. There were people like Helen Glover and Lizzy Yarnold, who wanted to be the best in the world at something, all over the country. And we were in a very privileged place at UK Sport, in that we were able to make some of those dreams come true.

Because I was still working for the YST, I was also able to link excellence with grassroots participation. There are lots of young people out there looking for excitement, wanting to be challenged and stretched, but the world had changed.

I used to get my adrenalin fix by roller-skating down Farm Road with Brian Carrier, and I lost count of the number of times I fell out of a tree. Back then, bruised elbows, grazed knees and the odd broken bone were just a normal part of growing up, but young people tend to interact less with the real world nowadays, and some choose to get their adventure and excitement from elsewhere.

One year, at our annual YST camp for developing young leaders, we included a group of teenagers, many of whom had been in trouble with the police. On the first day, they caused havoc and my team wanted to send them home. I told them to leave this group with me so I could provide them with a busier and more challenging programme of activity. One evening, we were due to have a quiz session but, reckoning this group might be disruptive, I sat with them watching football on TV instead. And when I asked the young man sitting next to me why he was in trouble, he told me he liked to steal cars.

'What's it like to steal a car?' I asked.

'Really exciting. You get this dry feeling in your mouth and your heart is going b'doink, b'doink, b'doink, almost bursting through your chest . . .'

He built up this scene, with a lot of swear words thrown in, and when he got to the end, I said, 'Wow, I know what you mean. I've felt like that.'

'What, you've stolen cars?'

'No, I haven't stolen any cars. But I have played sport for my country, so I know what you mean about your tongue sticking to the roof of your mouth—'

'That's right.'

'And your heart almost bursting through your chest, when normally you don't even think about it—'

'Yeah! I didn't know you could get that feeling from anything else.'

Afterwards, I contacted a man I knew who ran an indoor climbing school nearby.

'I'm sending someone over tomorrow,' I said. 'Keep him safe but make it exciting and very scary.' The following evening, I was having tea in the canteen with about two hundred young people when this boy came over with a big smile on his face.

'Miss,' he said, 'it scared the life out of me – but I loved every minute.'

I have no idea what happened to him. Maybe he went back to stealing cars. But maybe being scared witless on a climbing wall sparked something inside him and he started down a different path. I do hope so.

Through Sky Sports Living for Sport, which was launched in partnership with the YST and lasted for fourteen years, Olympic and Paralympic athletes were trained to work with thousands of disadvantaged young people who had lost their way and were in need of some inspiration. It was a great example of athletes giving back, reinvesting in their sport and young people, rather than disappearing off into the sunset with their medals.

One Living for Sport mentor who stood out was Steve Brown, captain of GB's wheelchair rugby team. Steve came to one of my YST youth camps, and gave an inspirational talk one evening. He explained that when he was their age, he was able-bodied and living life to the full. He was working as an area manager for a holiday company in Cologne and hoping to be promoted. Then one day, while Steve was standing on a balcony, he slipped and fell backwards over the railing, plunged down twelve feet and broke his neck. As Steve told his story, the audience sat there, open-mouthed.

After surgery in Germany, Steve was transferred to Stoke Mandeville Hospital, home to the National Spinal Injuries Centre. When he was told he'd never walk again, he felt that there was no point in living. But about a month after his accident, a physiotherapist took him to watch the GB wheelchair rugby team. He was transfixed by these men, some of them with worse injuries than him, trying to knock each other out of their wheelchairs, while shouting, swearing and bickering. 'If they can do that,' thought Steve, 'then why can't I?'

Less than five months after breaking his neck, Steve attended his first wheelchair rugby training session. Within a year, he was in the GB squad, and narrowly missed out on selection for the 2008 Olympics. And in 2011, he was appointed captain. At this point in his story, all these tough teenagers stood up and started clapping. Some of them had tears running down their faces. When they'd finally quietened down, Steve said: 'Let me leave you with one really important message – why did I have to lose the use of two-thirds of my body before I decided to make the most of the one-third I had left? Don't make the same mistake.' Steve is one of the most charming, gentle, sweet guys you could meet, but his story and its message has an impact like a sledgehammer.

While too many people underestimate how much sport can bring to young people's lives – the thrill it can provide, the sense of purpose – it can also leave a gaping hole when people who have made a career out of sport are forced to retire and enter the normal world. Having spent almost every day training to be the best they can possibly be, they no longer have a goal. And nothing in the normal world can match the highs of competing.

It was Tessa Jowell's idea to make Kelly Holmes the first 'school sport champion' in 2006, with a remit to visit schools and inspire and motivate children. A talented schoolgirl runner, Kelly joined the Army at eighteen and became a physical training instructor. She returned to athletics full time in 1997, and it was a long, often painful journey to Olympic glory. Having won two World Championships silver medals and a bronze at the 2000 Olympics, she injured herself in 2003, before falling into a depression. But she fought her way back to full fitness and won two gold medals at the 2004 Olympics, before retiring the following year.

When I started working with Kelly, she was eager to find a new purpose. She'd spent two decades working towards a goal, and since she'd won those two gold medals in Athens – which is about as high as it was possible to go – she'd been groping in the dark, trying to find a replacement goal and some kind of meaning. She did a terrific job as school sport champion, inspiring thousands of young people and working tirelessly to give back to sport. Eventually she was clear about her own mission and launched her own charity, the Dame Kelly Holmes Trust, in 2008, while also becoming a sought-after motivational speaker and mental health advocate.

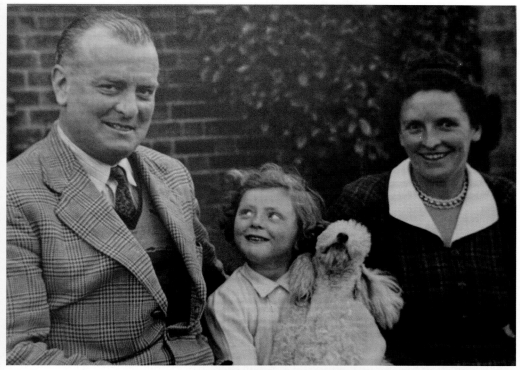

(above) My wonderful parents Robert and Pat Campbell with Charlie the dog – the adoring look at my dad says it all.

(right) Sister Gill and Charlie the dog – our childhood was full of laughter and happy memories.

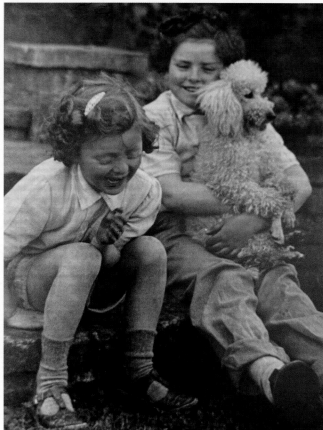

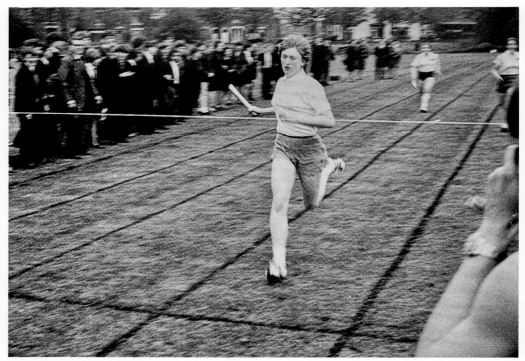

Winning the relay race for my house team at school sports day. My time at Long Eaton Grammar school shaped my sporting life.

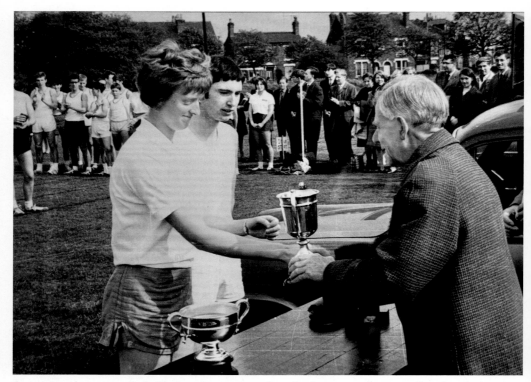

Receiving the cup on behalf of my house team for winning sports day, as well as the *victrix ludorum* for achieving the most individual points.

Playing goal defence for school, college, club and country gave me great joy, lifelong friendships and special memories.

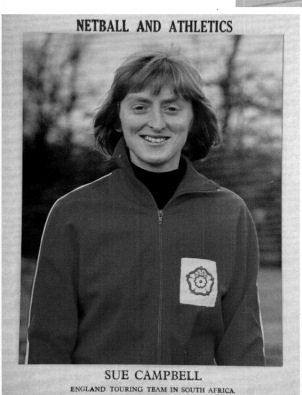

NETBALL AND ATHLETICS

SUE CAMPBELL

ENGLAND TOURING TEAM IN SOUTH AFRICA.
1973
ENGLAND ATHLETIC TEAM

Pulling on an England shirt to represent your country is the proudest moment any sportsman or woman can have.

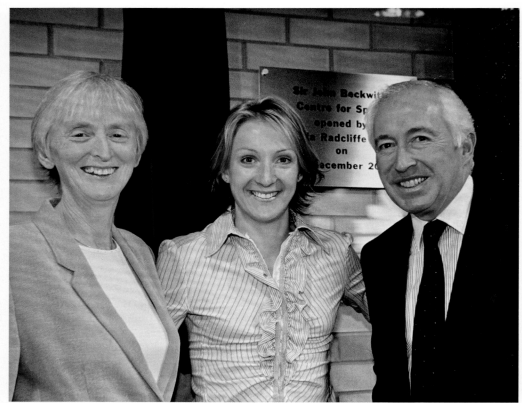

(above) Opening the new Sir John Beckwith Centre at Loughborough University with Youth Sport Trust founder Sir John and Paula Radcliffe.

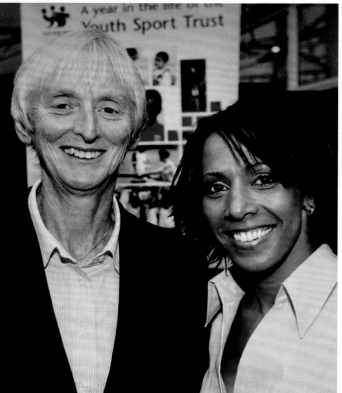

(left) After winning two gold medals at the 2004 Olympics, Dame Kelly Holmes became the National School Sport Champion on behalf of the YST.

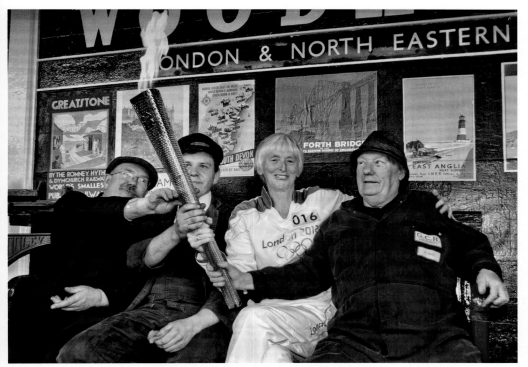

A special day as I collect the London Olympic torch at the local Quorn and Woodhouse railway station and run through my village surrounded by people cheering all the way.

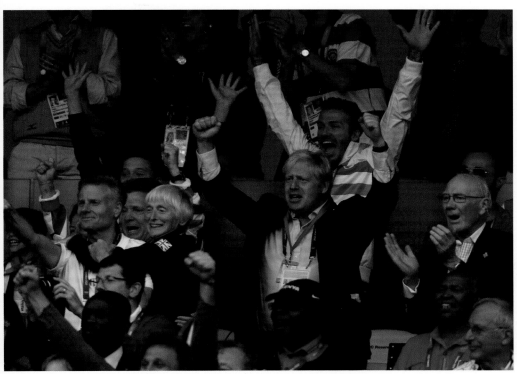

Celebrating another Olympic gold with Lord Paul Deighton (Chief Executive of London 2012), Boris Johnson (then Mayor of London) and David Beckham. *(Alexander Hassenstein/Getty Images)*

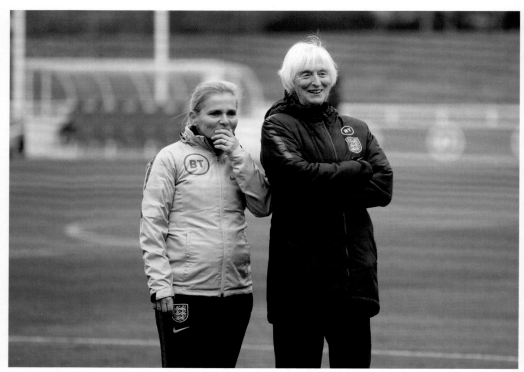

England women's coach Sarina Wiegman and I watching the squad train at St George's Park, the home of the men's, women's and para England teams. *(Naomi Baker/Getty Images)*

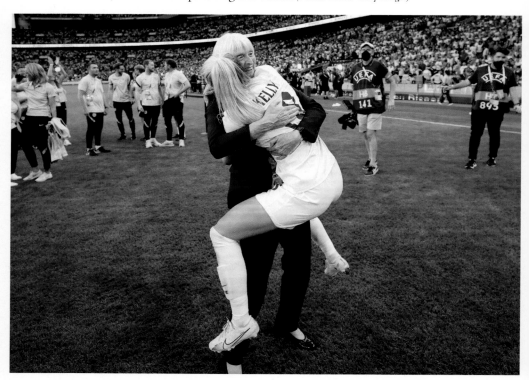

Pure joy! Chloe Kelly and I embrace after England win Euro 2022 at Wembley in front of 87,000 people, with 17 million watching on television. *(Lynne Cameron - The FA/Getty Images)*

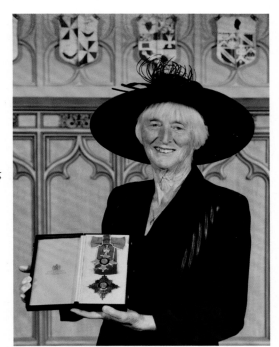

A very proud day at Windsor Castle, receiving my DBE for services to sport.

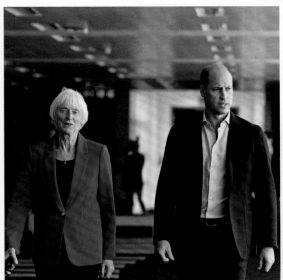

Accompanying the Prince of Wales to meet the England players at St George's Park prior to Euro 2022.
(PAUL ELLIS/Getty Images)

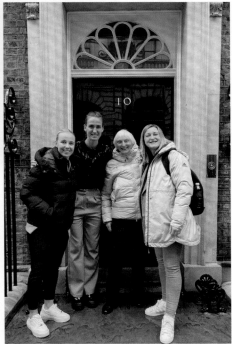

Beth Mead, Ellen White and Jill Scott join me at Number 10 to hear Prime Minister Rishi Sunak confirm the investment in school sport the Lionesses asked for after the Euros was going to be delivered.

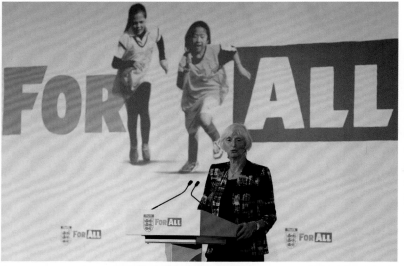

Speaking passionately about football being accessible and welcoming for everyone as players, coaches, referees and administrators at every level of the game. *(Matt Lewis – The FA/Getty Images)*

Denise Lewis and Jill Scott presenting me with the British Sport Industry Lifetime Achievement Award – a special moment for me and everyone who has worked alongside me over the years. *(Anthony Harvey/Shutterstock for Sport industry Awards)*

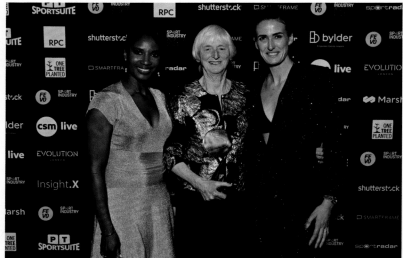

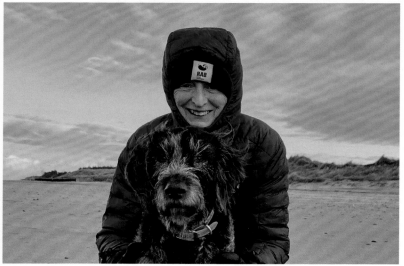

My wonderful companion and friend Willow and I on our favourite beach in Norfolk on a blustery autumn day.

10

Dealing with the tough times

Try not to take things personally, remember
the mission and get back on track

Gordon Brown replaced Tony Blair as Prime Minister in June 2007, and while I'm not sure he saw sport as a vehicle for social change in the same way as Tony did, he respected sport and was enthusiastic about the Olympic project.

Before the 2008 Olympics in Beijing, Gordon Brown asked me to set up two sports initiatives to tie in with Seb's promise to bring sport to children all over the world. At UK Sport we had already set up International Inspiration under the outstanding leadership of Debbie Lye (a former DCMS civil servant). We were working in partnership with UNICEF, the British Council and the YST to drive our ambition to reach twenty countries around the world to use sport to inspire twelve million children. Each project was created in consultation with the policy makers and designed to drive social change

— tackling social cohesion in Brazil, improving PE in India, using sport to open education on HIV and AIDS in Zambia, teaching swimming in Bangladesh or training sports leaders in Ethiopia. It was the 'sport for all' policy we had spoken about so many times in the UK which had so often fallen on deaf ears.

So when Gordon Brown asked me for two sports initiatives, one in India was already up and running but the other, in China (not involved in International Inspiration), required a bit of work. So off we went with Gordon and Sarah Brown on a whistle-stop trip to China and India. I went on several visits with Sarah and found her to be a compassionate and caring woman and someone whose company I enjoyed. The contrived table-tennis event we set up in China seemed to go down well, after which off we went to India.

The 'Magic Bus' was one of a number of schemes in India and it involved the bus travelling to villages and providing young people with the opportunity to get active and play sport. The focus was on giving girls and young women the self-confidence and self-esteem to play a full part in society through engagement in sport. On the plane home, the PM showed me a big photo album the Indian Government had given him, including a great snap of him and the Magic Bus children. 'Isn't this a fabulous picture?' he said, with a big grin on his face. He was genuinely delighted with the work we were doing.

★   ★   ★

Around the same time, I was doing a young people's event in the garden of Number 10. After the PM had finished playing rugby with the children, he took me aside and said, 'Did you know they want to offer you a peerage and put you in the House of Lords?' The House of Lords Commission did a regular check to see if all areas of government policy were covered by the existing members and had felt there was the need for additional sport policy expertise. I had been invited to a 'discussion' but had heard nothing since, so his question was confirmation that I had clearly passed the test. I hesitated and said I appreciated it was a great honour but I needed to give it further thought because of all my other commitments. In discussion with a few key confidants I decided that this would give me a platform to advocate the case for sport, so in 2008 I accepted and entered the House of Lords. My parents would never have believed it!

Pete Keen had always said that it takes six to eight years to build a fully functioning performance system, and we'd only just started on the journey with some of the sports. But despite UK Sport having predicted that Team GB would finish eighth in the medal table at the 2008 Olympics in Beijing, we finished fourth, winning forty-seven medals instead of the expected thirty-five, nineteen of them gold (we ended up with fifty-one medals, after Russia were stripped of four because of doping violations). That was the most gold medals Britain had won since the London Games of 1908 and had us wondering if we should recalibrate and target third in 2012.

It was more difficult to predict how many Paralympic medals we'd win in Beijing because, prior to the 2004 Olympics, Paralympic sport, in the UK and elsewhere, had been a mix of élite performance and participation.

To achieve an Olympic medal, an athlete had to be in the talent confirmation system for at least six years (although there were outliers), but Paralympic athletes had a less structured International competitive programme in those days and often prepared one or two years ahead of the Paralympics. As such, Paralympic athletes required a completely different funding formula.

By 2008, we were doing a better job investing in Paralympic medal prospects but still hadn't got the individual sports' talent pathways sorted. Athletes we put on talent pathways would come to the fore at London 2012. UK Sport identified ninety-five medals we expected to win in Beijing, including thirty-five golds, to finish second in the table. And as with the Olympics, we overperformed, winning 102 medals, including forty-two golds (seven more than we won in 2004), to finish behind only China.

The following year, I made my maiden speech in the House of Lords. I spoke about my work with the YST, how PE and sport were helping improve academic standards and behaviour, even in the most challenging schools. I spoke about the positive impact PE and sport could have on health and well-being, and how they were helping tackle issues of social inclusion and community cohesion. I spoke about my hope that a home Olympics would consolidate PE and sport's place at the heart of every school. PE and sport, I argued, weren't just games, they were a way of building a new youth culture.

The school sport system the YST had built, in conjunction with the Labour Government, was indeed the envy of countries all over the world. And in 2008, the PE & Sport Strategy for Young People was launched, to build upon the existing approach. Supported by funding of £755 million, to be spent between 2008 and 2011, the purpose of the new strategy was to continue increasing the percentage of children doing two hours of high-quality sport a week and create opportunities for children to participate in a further three hours a week. It was a case of onwards and upwards – and then the Coalition Government (Conservative and Lib Dem) came into power.

On 20 October 2010, Education Secretary Michael Gove wrote to tell me that the Coalition Government planned to remove all ring-fenced funding for School Sport Partnerships, phase out specialist sports colleges and dismantle the existing PE and school sport strategy. In his letter, he said that not enough pupils were playing competitive sport and that his plan was to implement an 'Olympic-style approach to school sport'. There was no more detail than that.

When the government went public with its plans, there was a massive national outcry. Andy Burnham pointed out that his predecessor as shadow Education Secretary, Mr Gove's fellow Tory Hugh Robertson, had praised School Sport Partnerships as a success and promised that his party would build on them. Journalists from across the political spectrum reacted with bemusement. Five years earlier, Seb Coe had told the world that a London Olympics would inspire a generation of children, and now, barely two years before the event, Mr Gove had taken a sledgehammer to PE and school sport in the UK.

From the moment Sir John Beckwith gave me the opportunity to work with the YST, we'd worked so hard to build an incredible system that embedded PE and sport into every school in the country. There were three thousand people working in PE and school sport as part of a national framework. We had created an exciting, optimistic legacy which was the envy of the world. And now it was being dismantled. It was all so brutal and cruel, one of the biggest acts of vandalism ever to have happened to sport in British schools. And one from which we have never recovered!

I had people ringing me from all over the country, asking me to intervene. Mr Gove did meet me but was adamant that the whole programme would end. I produced statistics and data to show the impact on school standards, physical activity levels and the growth of school club links for our most talented young people, but he was not for turning. I was reduced to pleading with anyone who would listen to me – civil servants, special advisors, ministers – to stop this decision. I tried to get across the insanity of destroying a much-lauded PE and school sport system two years before the London Olympics. I explained that we'd have to make as many as three thousand people redundant. I tried everything

I had learned from years of working with politicians. But nobody could do anything. Before then, I'd almost always been able to persuade people of the transformative power of sport, but Mr Gove didn't seem to understand it and didn't want to be a part of it.

It was deeply depressing, traumatic and hurtful – the lowest point of my professional career. I vividly remember walking up Whitehall crying my eyes out. The pain I felt is difficult to describe, other than to say it was physical. I felt like I'd spent thirteen years building my perfect home – brick by brick, floor by floor – only for someone to come along and set fire to it, while my hands were tied behind my back, so that I could only watch it burn to the ground.

Mercifully, Sir John Beckwith had always been a kind and generous man. And now I had to ring him and say, 'Sir John, I really need a lot of help. I don't want one person to leave the YST without a job, help with their CVs and some financial support. But I can't afford to do it, because Mr Gove has taken a great deal of our money away.' Sir John told me to do what I needed, and that he would ensure we were not out of pocket.

I ended up having to let go more than 50 per cent of my YST colleagues, people who had always given me their very best and done nothing wrong. Some of them sat in front of me and cried, told me they'd work for nothing, and I had to tell them I couldn't let them do that. Many of them went on to do great things elsewhere, but it was a heart-breaking process. My number two Steve Grainger, who had been with me since the National Coaching Foundation, told me he couldn't go back to the beginning and start all over again. I replied, 'I don't blame you in the slightest.' In 2011, Steve joined the Rugby Football Union as director of development, working for John Steele, and he's still working there.

I'd been the mission leader for the school sport movement, always clear about the direction of travel, but now I had lost my way. Had I not been chair of UK Sport, working for them a few days a week, I'd have been in an even worse state. I stopped taking calls about anything to do with the demise of the network. I had done everything in my power to stop the vandalism, to no avail, and I could no longer bear the pain of desperate people's voices. I even wondered if I should wrap up the YST. Our core money had been taken away, the mission we had been on since 1995 had been blown out of the water, thousands had been made redundant. 'What,' I asked, 'is the point of it all?'

Then one day, my PA said she'd received a call that I had to take. It was from a sixteen-year-old girl, Debbie Foote, who had been on one of our youth leadership courses. Debbie started talking about how wrong it all was and how she was going to do something about it, and I responded with something along the lines of, 'That's terrific, Debbie, thank you,' before bringing the conversation to an end. I wasn't very communicative at the time.

A few weeks later, Debbie phoned me again. She told me she'd gathered 750,000 signatures and organised for young people to deliver the petition to Downing Street. Then she asked if I'd meet them somewhere outside the Houses of Parliament once they were finished. What followed was one of those incredible moments that brought me back to my mission.

The first thing I saw was this big crowd of young people marching down Whitehall, before turning right into Downing Street. Once they'd handed in their petition they headed south again, to the sound of taxi drivers tooting their horns. Then they crossed the green where I was waiting and engulfed me. They were all wearing T-shirts that said, 'DON'T CUT SCHOOL SPORT', and I thought, 'Sue Campbell, just remember that your mission has always been to help young people find their self-belief and confidence to take action through sport – and here they are, doing exactly that. You've always believed that sport can change lives – don't give up on it.' It took a sixteen-year-old girl to remind me of my moral purpose and give me a sharp reminder that whatever happens to you personally the mission you believe in carries on!

Afterwards, I went back to my beleaguered colleagues at the YST and showed them a video of a ship being tossed hither and thither by massive waves. And while they were watching, I asked three questions, as if I was the captain of the ship, and answered them myself. 'Can our ship survive this storm? Yes, it can because our ship was built on brilliant values, with a strong moral purpose that cannot be broken. How many crew are we going to lose? Well, we've sadly lost a lot already – but you're still on this ship because we need you to lift your heads and drive this ship forward. And finally, where on earth are we heading? I can't answer that right now, but together we'll find a way.'

Sport is my passion and my purpose. I love it dearly. It speaks to me, and I've been blessed in that I've been able to make it speak for other people, whether by improving their day-to-day lives or helping make their dreams come true. So, my resilience comes from knowing my purpose and being stubbornly unwilling to turn my back on my mission. If the YST really had to reinvent itself, so be it.

At the time, the Coalition Government's Secretary of State for Culture, Media and Sport was Jeremy Hunt, who was also Minister for the Olympics. Jeremy was unable to make Mr Gove rethink his decision, despite my pleading, but he did tell me he wanted to take a look at how these School Sport Partnerships worked. And when he returned from his visits, he waxed lyrical about how incredible they were and what a dedicated and committed group of people he had met. Then he said, 'Is there any way you can salvage any of it?'

As difficult as it was to accept that thirteen years' work had been wiped out, this might be an opportunity for some of the great network of people to survive and start a slow rebuild programme. The YST had been running the School Games National Finals (the brainchild of Richard Caborn), where the best school-age youngsters from England, Wales, Northern Ireland and Scotland competed in a number of sports – athletics, swimming, table tennis, badminton, volleyball and so on. It was an inclusive competition with events for disabled competitors. Ellie Simmonds and Hannah Cockroft were among the early champions. Jeremy wanted to know if we could expand the School Games across the School Sport Partnership network and create a four-tier competition in England: intra-school, inter-school, county and then the national finals. The network was in the process of being dismantled but could we create School Games Organisers (SGOs) to coordinate local provision across School Sport Partnerships. This would give the 450 partnership development managers a lifeline. The only challenge was funding. In the end Jeremy asked Sport England to consider funding these posts and also went to the Secretary of State for Health to see if he could persuade them to invest. Eventually we had just enough money (£7 million) to fund the SGOs for three days a week. That network still exists and many of the old partnership development managers are still involved thanks to their resilience, determination and passion.

Politics can be so divisive and people become very partisan: they are either left or right. But in reality it is down to individuals, regardless of their party affiliation, and there are conviction politicians on all sides. While it's true that Tony Blair and Gordon Brown's governments understood the benefits of PE and school sport far better than their Tory successors, Jeremy Hunt was incredibly good to me and to school sport at a very difficult time.

Jeremy is from a very different background to me, having attended private school and Oxford University, but we found common ground and developed a very close relationship. He was always quick to pick up the phone or reply to texts, because he wanted to help. And while he couldn't persuade Michael Gove to change his mind – and I genuinely believe he tried – he found a way to move forward. So while the school sport structure that we built was still decimated, thanks to Jeremy's intervention we managed to retain some of it. Without him, school sport would be in an even worse place, if such a thing is possible.

Fast-forward to 4 August 2012, and what became known as 'Super Saturday' – that incredible evening in London when Jess Ennis, Greg Rutherford and Mo Farah all won Olympic gold for Great Britain in the space of forty-four minutes.

I was in the VIP area of the Olympic Stadium, meeting and greeting the various VIPs, wearing my GB tracksuit. Jeremy and his wife were there and we began talking about the heptathlon and how Jess could win the gold even if she didn't win the 800m race. Jeremy's wife found this a difficult concept and I was invited to sit with her to talk her through the race. In the end I didn't need to explain anything, as Jess won the race and her well-deserved hard-earned gold medal. When Seb had to leave his seat to present Jess's medal, it left a space next to the Prime Minister David Cameron and Mayor of London Boris Johnson. Someone asked Jeremy to step in, but he suggested I go instead. I told him I couldn't possibly sit next to the PM and the Mayor of London while wearing a tracksuit, but he insisted, sending me off with the line, 'Make sure you tell the PM about school sport.'

I've still got the picture of me sitting with Mr Cameron and Mr Johnson. What it doesn't show is me bending Mr Cameron's ear, which is what I did the whole time Mo Farah was running his 10,000m. We then all celebrated with hugs as Mo crossed the line, completing one of the most remarkable nights in athletics history.

By the time the evening was over I had convinced the PM to secure the funding for the Rio Olympics and Paralympics and started a conversation about resurrecting school sport. It was clear that there could be no going back, so what could be done?

I told him that if I had funding I would put it all into primary schools. I explained that if you don't embed physical activity in children's daily lives by the time they're eleven, they're unlikely to suddenly start doing it when they reach secondary school. Mr Cameron asked me to describe what I had in mind, practically speaking. I talked him through the need for investment in teacher training, resources and support for primary teachers. He said he liked the idea and asked me to go to speak to Michael Gove about it. I didn't reply. Then Mr Cameron said, 'I'm asking you as your Prime Minister. Speak to him.'

So a few days later, I went to see Mr Gove in his office and gave him the same outline I had presented to the PM.

I described the various challenges primary-school children faced and all the different ways PE and sport could help. I reminded him that we had a growing obesity crisis on our hands costing the NHS billions, and explained that school improvement, attendance and pupil behaviour would all be positively impacted by a high-quality PE and sport curriculum. We needed investment in the professional development of teachers and resources to support them, plus improved facilities in many schools. As I was speaking, he raised his hand to stop me and said, 'I know the answer to this.'

'Do you, Sir?' I replied. "What's that?"

'Cups and trophies.'

I leaned forward and said, 'Can I just check that your strategic response to this major national issue for children's health and well-being is "cups and trophies"?'

'Yes.'

'No! That simply will not work.'

With that, Mr Gove looked at me and said, 'This conversation is finished.'

There was no point in me saying anything else anyway because it was abundantly clear that Mr Gove wasn't willing or able to understand the issues.

I assume Mr Gove meant that if there were cups and trophies children would play. The fact that a lot of children did not have anybody to teach them how to play sport or take them to events apparently hadn't occurred to him.

Once again, I found myself walking up Whitehall in despair. This was in the middle of the Olympics, and Great Britain was winning stacks of medals. I should have been happier than I'd ever been, but I was beyond distraught. As tough as it was going to be, it was time to go back to the drawing board and rebuild the school sport plan.

11

Resetting the bar

Be unafraid to reach higher and build
a vision that excites everyone

I needed to rewind again, because my meeting with Mr Gove was an unfortunate blip in an otherwise glorious month. The London Olympics and Paralympics seem like a long time ago now, but I will never forget those incredible moments and the joy the whole event brought to everyone across the UK.

Not everything went to plan, because nothing ever does, however meticulous you've been. And you don't get more meticulous than Pete Keen and Liz Nicholl.

For the best part of a decade, Pete and Liz tracked the progress of every potential British athlete and medal winner in London. Every single competition at European or World level, at almost every age group, was on their radar. And while it wasn't their job to tell the governing bodies what to do, they had provided the guidance and structure to maximise their potential.

UK Sport also did a quarterly open house with the media, at which we showed where each sport was in terms of governance, athlete preparation and performance system. We gave each sport a red, amber or green grade, which they were anxious about initially, but we thought it was important. Red meant that the sport was not meeting any of its targets, amber indicated some areas were being delivered but others still needed work and green meant the sport was on track with all aspects of their performance plan.

We were using public money, so needed to show we were heading in the right direction. As time went on, most of the sports changed from red to amber to green. And on the eve of London 2012, there were only a couple of sports left on amber.

I really believed in everything UK Sport and the governing bodies had done, and I trusted that all the investment would pay dividends. However, I did have a few wobbles in the days leading up to the opening ceremony.

We'd spent millions of pounds of public money and set ourselves an ambitious and very public medal target, and now we were about to reveal the results of our endeavours to the world. I remember Seb saying to me, 'This is going to be an amazing Olympics,' and me replying, 'The facilities are incredible and I don't doubt the organisation will be world class, but if we don't win lots of medals people may think we have failed!'

There was some nervousness in the media that the opening ceremony wouldn't be a patch on Beijing's spectacular effort four years earlier, but London 2012's exceeded all expectations, despite it costing less than half as much. Director Danny Boyle somehow managed to blend the Industrial Revolution, the NHS, the best of British literature, comedy, radio, TV and film – and much, much more – with British music ranging from classical to brass band to rock to electronic. Then of course there was that quite brilliant film of HM The Queen meeting James Bond at Buckingham Palace, the two of them apparently climbing into a helicopter together and parachuting into the stadium. I'm not sure a host nation will ever be able to top that moment. Pure genius.

But I must say my favourite part of the opening ceremony was the lighting of the Olympic cauldron. While it's often lit by a top athlete, most famously by Muhammad Ali at Atlanta 1996, this time the torch was carried into the stadium by five-time Olympic champion Steve Redgrave, who then passed it on to a team of seven youngsters. The youngsters jogged a lap before being greeted by seven great British Olympians – Steve, Daley Thompson, Kelly Holmes, Mary Peters, Lynn Davies, Duncan Goodhew, Shirley Robertson – and each presented with a torch. Flanked by 260 British Olympic medallists, the youngsters made their way to the centre of the stadium, lit some of the 206 copper petals (each one was inscribed with the name of a participating nation) and watched as the flames spread and then rose to light the cauldron. At that moment, those two worlds of mine – sporting excellence and sport as a vehicle to empower young people – became one. It felt so personal and so real.

I returned to my hotel that night almost bursting with pride, because we'd put on one hell of a show for the world. However, the next few days didn't go to plan . . . At least not as far as the results were concerned.

We had hoped that the men's cyclists would get us off to a flying start in the road race – Mark Cavendish, the reigning world champion, was backed by a dream team that included Bradley Wiggins, who had just won the Tour de France, and Chris Froome, who would win the Tour the following year – but they all finished well out of the medals. When we still hadn't won a gold after four days of competition, colleagues were ringing me up in a state of high anxiety. And journalists were sharpening their knives, ready to write mocking articles about how hubristic and ridiculous our target of sixty-five medals had been.

Then, on 1 August, the dam finally burst. And who won Great Britain's first gold of the 2012 Olympics? Helen Glover and Heather Stanning, who were both products of our talent identification programme. Later that day, Bradley Wiggins won gold in the time trial, and after that the medals started pouring in.

While our athletes were doing their thing, my role was to be anywhere and everywhere, because I needed to persuade as many influential people as possible that the London Games weren't a full stop but a platform on which to build even bigger and better. But it was also about soaking up the atmosphere and enjoying the success of our sportsmen and -women.

Super Saturday will forever be etched on my mind, as it will be for the other eighty thousand people who were in the Olympic Stadium that evening. Whenever I think of Jess Ennis winning the 800m to clinch heptathlon gold – flinging her head back and arms wide as she crosses the finish line – my skin tingles. And while I was bugging the PM for most of Mo Farah's 10,000m, I did have the sense to shut up for the final couple of laps, so I can still picture that too! We won six gold medals that day (two more in rowing and one in cycling), to make it our most successful since the 1908 Games.

Other highlights of the Games were being in the velodrome when Chris Hoy won the keirin to become the most successful British Olympian in history (the place went completely bonkers!) and watching rower Katherine Grainger finally win gold, alongside Anna Watkins, after three successive silvers. But sometimes it's the simple things that stay with you the longest.

Liz Nicholl and I were staying in a hotel near Regent's Park, and we'd ring each other on the way back there every evening. We would talk about that day's successes before deciding who was going to pick up a bottle of white wine and a bag of crisps, which we'd share while watching the review of the day's action on the BBC. Having been on this incredible journey together, there was something perfect about those evenings watching things unfold so beautifully, and I know she thought the same. Even today, if you mention me and the Olympics to Liz, there's a good chance she'll say, 'White wine and crisps.'

Another moment that stands out is walking over the bridge in the Olympic Park and seeing hundreds of people standing on the grass banks, watching a British athlete being awarded their gold medal on the big screen and belting out the national anthem. I can't remember which athlete it was, but that wasn't important. What was important was the diversity of the people singing the anthem. They were people of all ages, all cultures, and no doubt all classes and religions, and they brought a tear to my eye. I thought to myself, 'This is more than just sport – this is unashamed pride in our nation.'

Modern Britain is one of the most diverse countries on earth, and there are more and more people asking, 'What does it mean to be British today? What binds the country together?' Sport isn't the only answer, but it is one of them, because British sporting success can give people a sense of belonging and pride and make them feel part of something bigger than themselves.

Nelson Mandela said it best, with a quote that has inspired me every day since I first heard it:

'Sport has the power to change the world. It has the power to inspire. It has the power to unite people in a way that little else does. It speaks to youth in a language they understand. Sport can create hope where once there was only despair. It is more powerful than government in breaking down racial barriers.'

I'm certain the people I saw in the Olympic Park that day went home feeling more optimistic about being part of this country. And even if they weren't touched that deeply, they at least went home happier.

A Britain that was almost apologetic about winning – 'Let's give it a good try, chaps, and see what happens' – had been replaced by a Britain that was revelling in the fact that its athletes were winning medals by the bucketload. Everyone had stories about how the Games improved the mood of London: how everyone in the city suddenly seemed more friendly; how taxi drivers wanted to discuss dressage or diving; how even people on the Tube were talking to and smiling at each other. I recall the BBC's athletics presenter Gabby Logan describing how she returned home late one night, after another thrilling day in the Olympic Stadium, collapsed on the sofa with her husband and a gin and tonic and thought, 'I've never been happier in my life.' I think that was true of a lot of people that fortnight. What price do you put on that?

No business plan has ever delivered everything it said it would – but amazingly Pete Keen's did, and he'd written it six years ahead of time. Having predicted Team GB would win sixty-five medals, that's exactly what they did. Pete didn't get every sport's performance bang on – a couple, like swimming, fell short of expectations, while a few exceeded them – and we finished third in the medal table, not fourth. But I don't remember anyone complaining.

As for gymnastics, having slashed its budget and decided to invest most of the money in Beth Tweddle and a group

of lads who were showing promise as juniors, it contributed a barely believable four medals – a bronze from Beth
in the women's uneven bars, silver and bronze from Louis
Smith and Max Whitlock in the pommel horse, and bronze
in the men's artistic team all-around. That equalled Great
Britain's tally from all previous Games combined (we'd
won one medal since 1928 before then, Louis Smith's
bronze in 2008).

For most of its modern history, gymnastics had been a
sport that the United States, China and Eastern European
countries won medals in, and hardly anyone else. But now
we were a player – who'd have thought it?

After Beth and the men's success, I found Alan Sommerville,
who was now chair of British gymnastics, shedding tears of
joy in the stands. He gave me the biggest hug, before pushing me away and saying, 'Now give me your money!' just as
he'd promised to do nine years earlier, when I'd informed
him that we were drastically cutting his beloved sport's funding. 'Sure will!' I replied.

If our strategy of focusing on a small pool of talent looked
hard-nosed at the time, it had proved better than spreading
ourselves too thin and coming up with nothing. And if
British Gymnastics could mould a group of talented youngsters into world-class Olympians once, they could surely do
it again.

While the final day of London 2012 was mainly about
celebrating a job very well done, I was still bending David
Cameron's ear. And probably around the time that Anthony

Joshua was winning Great Britain's twenty-ninth and final gold medal of the Games in the boxing ring, Mr Cameron was assuring me that the investment would be retained through to Rio 2016. On reflection, that was probably my biggest achievement of the Olympic fortnight, because it meant that UK Sport would not have to waste time and energy arguing for investment and sports could start fine-tuning for Rio almost as soon as London was over.

That pride I'd felt during the Olympics – in the spectacular show that London was putting on for the rest of the world, in our athletes, our fans, our organisers, our volunteers, our country as a whole – grew even more intense when the Paralympics came to town a little over two weeks later.

Too often the Paralympics has an 'after the Lord Mayor's show' feel about it, but that certainly wasn't the case in London. More than four thousand athletes from 164 countries participated, which was eighteen more than in Beijing 2008. There were even athletes from the Solomon Islands and North Korea.

Great Britain had the biggest team, with 294 athletes, and the public came out to support them in droves. More than 2.4 million advance tickets were sold (five times more than for Beijing) and venues were packed for all ten days of competition. There was wall-to-wall coverage on Channel 4 and there were front-page headlines in most of the newspapers (in America, rights-holding network NBC broadcast almost nothing of the Paralympics).

The view of the Paralympians had changed for good. No longer was it a case of, 'Wow, isn't it wonderful how these disabled people can do sport' but rather 'These are élite sportspeople with a disability.' People saw them as serious athletes, striving for glory on the world stage in exactly the same way as a Jess Ennis or a Mo Farah. People were no longer embarrassed around disability: they were in awe of it. The *Guardian* journalist Jonathan Freedland said it best in an article published in September 2012: 'If, say, an amputee in team colours went by in a wheelchair [in the Olympic Park], heads would turn. Not because they were staring at someone with a disability, but in case they'd spotted a Paralympic celebrity. They didn't want to stare, they wanted an autograph.'

It was impossible not to be open-mouthed watching some of the feats on display. I'll never forget seeing a Brazilian high-jumper with one leg. Having walked to his mark on two crutches, he discarded one of them, which brought a round of applause. He then discarded the other, which brought a bigger round of applause, and had me thinking, 'How does this work then?' He then steadied himself for three or four seconds, before hopping towards the bar and clearing it. Cue pandemonium in the stadium. And that wasn't a patronising response, that was just people recognising that they were watching something very special.

I travelled on the Tube every day, and the conversations I heard were so uplifting. The language around disability had changed, in that there was very little mention of impairments. Instead, people were excited to watch great sport performed by world-class athletes. And it didn't get any better than 'Thriller Thursday', that unforgettable evening in the Olympic Stadium when Hannah Cockroft, David Weir and Jonnie Peacock all won gold for Team GB.

Great Britain finished third in the medal table, behind China and Russia (we'd finished second at Beijing 2008 but actually won eighteen more medals in London). Wheelchair athlete David Weir and cyclist Sarah Storey won four gold medals each to become household names, along with Hannah Cockroft (two golds), Jonnie Peacock (who beat Paralympic legend Oscar Pistorius in the 100m for athletes with a single below-knee amputation) and swimmer Ellie Simmonds (two golds, a silver and a bronze).

Seb said in his closing speech, 'We will never think of disability sport in the same way,' and I think he was right. But did we do enough to keep that mood alive? I'm not so sure. For while those mesmerising ten days of competition made superstars of a handful of athletes and changed many people's attitudes towards disabled people, research shows that disabled sportspeople do not get the access, opportunities or investment afforded to able-bodied sportspeople.

While UK Sport has increased funding for élite Paralympic sport, research suggests that London 2012 had a minimal impact on the number of disabled people taking part in sport. Before you create inspiration, which the London Paralympic Games did, you have already to have built additional opportunities – real legacy only happens if you plan ahead, not after the event. You have to plan; it doesn't happen because you want it to. So while disability-specific sports clubs were geared up for an influx of new participants, most sports clubs didn't have the knowledge or resources to provide for disabled people.

When I told David Cameron about my meeting with Michael Gove and his 'cups and trophies' comment, he didn't sigh or roll his eyes. He was too much the consummate politician for that. Instead, he asked me to start working to come up with a new scheme for PE and sport in primary schools, which I was happy to do.

I was to work with Seb, who had been made Olympic legacy ambassador. Seb, of course, had made much of the London Games inspiring young people, but while I'm sure he was frustrated that the Coalition Government had seriously undermined his message, at least in the UK, I'm not sure he had time to get angry about it. Naturally, he'd been myopically focused on the whopping task of delivering the Olympics. But now the Games were over, he saw how devastating Mr Gove's measures would be (in a recent tribute to me, Seb referred to the 'maladroit ministers' who had undone my good work).

Seb, some hard-working civil servants and I came up with something called the PE and Sport Premium. As far as I was concerned, the idea was to invest in upskilling primary-school teachers, create good resources and a workable curriculum. Unfortunately, Mr Gove was responsible for the grants to primary schools but had no overarching strategy. The grants were made directly to head teachers, there was limited monitoring by Ofsted and no direct accountability for schools in terms of how the money was spent.

Some head teachers did a great job of making it work, but others spent the money on other things, which is the problem with the manner in which it was distributed. Not that I blamed them – if your roof is caving in and money is tight, you're going to fix the roof before thinking about PE and sport provision.

Some heads called in the 'white van men' as I labelled them. These were individuals (some good and some not so good) who were not trained teachers but had some sporting qualification and could offer a service. This would allow the teachers to spend time preparing for other lessons. What this achieved was the opposite of the ambition to upskill teachers in delivering physical education: it de-skilled teachers and left the PE lessons in the hands of others. But what did they know about teaching? Would a head bring in a random person to teach English or maths? Of course not. But because it was 'just' PE and sport, these people would do just fine.

It's not for me to comment on Michael Gove's overall legacy as Education Secretary, but he was one of many who failed to understand that children need a much more rounded education than we provide them with so that all their talents and skills can shine.

PE and school sport in the UK have never recovered since Mr Gove's intervention in 2010. By 2008, remember, 92 per cent of English young people were doing at least two hours of PE or sport a week. In 2022 a Sport England survey revealed that only 47 per cent of children were meeting the Chief Medical Officer's recommended daily activity level of at least sixty minutes. The number of PE teachers has fallen, and the hours of PE and sport being taught in secondary schools in England dropped from 326,000 hours in 2011–12 to 286,000 hours in 2022–3.

Ironically, schools are now getting three times more funding for PE and sport than when the Coalition Government came to power, mainly because of the 'sugar tax' that was introduced in 2018 (when Jeremy Hunt was Health Secretary). But money on its own isn't enough: it has to be embedded in a long-term strategy, with the right people running things – people who understand the importance of PE as an integral part of a child's education. (I should say that quite a few School Sport Partnerships survive to this day, despite having their money and staff taken away, which is a great credit to everyone involved.)

I feel passionately that we misunderstand what education is about. The moral purpose of schools has got lost and the focus has become the 'business' of passing exams, which may work for some, but does not work for many young people.

I recently stood in front of a thousand head teachers and asked them to close their eyes. Then I said, 'Can you remember the moment you decided to become a teacher?' And after a pause, I asked, 'Now, would anybody who woke up one morning and thought, "I want to become a teacher so that I can get children to pass exams" please stand up.' There was laughter, and of course everybody stayed seated.

I'm all for academic success for those who are academic, but a school curriculum should speak to every child – and what about those young people who have other skills in sport, music, acting, dance, art or craftsmanship?

Youngsters today are constantly bombarded on social media, which means that they are always comparing themselves to others. As such, I wonder if many of them know who or what they are really meant to be. I remember England football legend Jill Scott saying that she only felt like the real her, and the best her, when she was playing football, and I was the same. When I was playing sport, I wasn't naughty or disruptive, and I never got told off. For so many young people taking part in a wider curriculum is when they discover who they are and what they want to be.

So many young people are disengaged from education simply because *they* don't value what *we* want them to value. But as I learned while teaching at Whalley Range High School, some challenging, alienated and unhappy young people are actually remarkable if you can find their magic spark. I was once one of those children, staring out of the window during lessons, dreaming about kicking a football around and even one day playing for England. Were it not for PE and Sheila Bassett my teacher goodness knows where I would have ended up. As it was, I found something that was the ultimate expression of me, which is why I'm so passionate about it to this day.

Just as there are different kinds of intelligence, people learn in different ways, and my journey has been far more about people skills than academic qualifications. I'm blessed with the ability to get on with most people, whether it's the person cleaning the office or the Prime Minister. And I learned most of those people skills from my parents.

My mum and dad weren't worried about me passing every exam I took. They understood that exam results were only one measure of success and that I had other useful skills and passions. School life should be about teaching young people how to build relationships, testing not just their memories but also their ability to live with others, work with others, listen to others, lead and follow others, and generally live successfully in society. It should be about producing young people who are confident, assured, flexible thinkers who are good at making decisions. And while sport isn't the only way to improve these young people's health, well-being and social skills, it can certainly make a massive contribution

My time at Whalley Range High School made me realise how challenging some children's lives are and how little hope they have. But as Nelson Mandela said, 'Sport can create hope where once there was only despair.' Mandela understood the power of sport – as did Tony Blair – unlike many other politicians. It's hard for me to understand why more don't.

Look at it this way: if you bought a car, put the wrong petrol in it, never checked its oil and water or never took it for an MOT, it wouldn't run for very long. At least you could buy a new one, but we only get one body, which we inhabit our whole life. What's the point of getting loads of GCSEs and A-levels if your life expectancy is limited?

I'm not being alarmist. The Royal College of Paediatrics and Child Health recently described the obesity issue as 'one of the greatest threats' to children and society. Obesity is the biggest cause of preventable cancer and can also lead to diabetes, infertility, high blood pressure, high cholesterol, breathing problems, back problems, heart disease, stroke, liver disease, arthritis and osteoarthritis. It costs the NHS about £6.5 billion a year, so you could argue that it's not just killing too many people, it's also killing the NHS.

According to the NHS, about 23 per cent of English kids are obese by the time they leave primary school and a further 14 per cent are overweight. These are scary numbers, especially when you consider that about 80 per cent of children who are obese in their early teens will go on to be obese adults (and a record number of young people are being treated for eating disorders such as anorexia and bulimia).

I read somewhere that childhood is no longer 'play-based' but 'phone-based', and while academics are still arguing over how much the worldwide mental health crisis in children has been caused by smartphones, I do sometimes wonder: is roaming the streets, like we used to, really more dangerous than spending hours a day on the internet? And how much real-life enrichment are young people missing out on while they're immersed in social media?

I'm not even talking about making reluctant children play football or rugby or tennis – or encouraging them to roller-skate down main roads, like Brian Carrier and I used to do (and which no adult ever pointed out might be quite danger-ous), I'm just talking about getting them outside in the fresh air for half an hour. At least let them walk to school and back, instead of driving them. If you're frightened of them getting knocked over by a car, walk with them!

It's scary how everyday activity has been removed from so many people's lives. In previous generations, most adults did manual labour, which was often exhausting. Nowadays, lots of people are sat on their backsides all day staring at a screen – including me! I can't do much exercise now because my body has just about given up on me, but I try to move about as much as possible and still walk the dogs twice a day, for a total of two hours, setting a good pace and keeping a record of how many steps I've done every week.

I'll be out walking by twenty to seven (if it's winter, I'll take a torch) because I'm at my best first thing in the morn-ing, and there's no better time to think than when you're walking your dogs. If I've got a problem that needs solving, or I need to prepare for a difficult meeting, that's the perfect time to do it.

In June 2010, the head teacher of a primary school invited me to give a talk to their teachers on physical education. When I walked into the room, it was very noisy and I could feel the tension. It was coming up to exam time, and I got the sense that everyone thought they had better things to do.

It was a beautiful sunny day, so I said to them, 'Rather than spend the next hour talking about why PE is important, I'm going to open those doors and we're all going to walk around that field together.'

I asked them to walk at a pace that made them nearly out of breath, and not to talk about work. Off they went in pairs, and when they came back in, I said, 'Shall I tell you what I've noticed? When I first walked into this room, you sounded like geese honking at each other in a barn.' They laughed, and I added, 'But doesn't it feel peaceful now you've calmed down and are ready to listen?' Well, that's why children need physical activity. Adults too.

I did say one last thing: 'Think about getting a dog, because they have to be exercised and you'll feel better for walking them!' Afterwards, a few of the teachers wrote to me to say they'd bought a dog. Let's hope they've enjoyed lots of walks together since that day.

12

Challenging the status quo

New ideas are not always welcome, but
they are what drives progress

I would have loved to have stayed at UK Sport until the Rio Olympics in 2016, but the rules stated that I was only allowed to do two terms, and by 2013 I'd actually done two-and-a-half, because of my two years as reform chair between 2003 and 2005.

Still, the government wanted me to be involved in an analysis of results in the London Games and the next round of planning, which took place in autumn/winter 2012. While we had exceeded expectations at the Olympics, our results in Paralympic sport had started to slip, so we decided to invest more heavily in Para for Rio. That worked a treat, with Team GB finishing second in the medal table at the Rio Paralympics with 147, 64 of them gold. That was twenty-seven more medals than London 2012 and almost twice as many golds. Team GB finished behind the United

States but ahead of China. I don't think anybody really expected that to happen.

I'd always said that the test of how well we had done our job at UK Sport would be what happened after I left. If things started to fall apart, I would have to admit that I had not led as well as I had hoped. As it was, Rio – and the Tokyo Games in 2021, where we didn't lose much ground – were testimony to the work everybody at UK Sport and the sports had done in building a sustainable high-performance system.

It hasn't been all plain sailing for UK Sport since my departure. There have been reports of coaches abusing athletes in several sports and continued criticism of UK Sport's overall philosophy, with some claiming that it is not holistic enough and too focused on winning medals – but we never advocated winning at all costs.

Coaches often tread a fine line between being necessarily tough and demanding high standards and making an athlete's life a misery. Any coach who is found to have abused athletes should be weeded out and called to account. All of us should put the health and well-being of our sportsmen and -women at the centre of all decisions we make.

The 'no compromise' approach has sometimes been misunderstood. It certainly did not mean treating athletes unfairly or abusing them physically or mentally. It meant providing athletes with the best support possible in all areas, which is costly and requires a focused use of funds. This does mean disappointing some sports and can be seen as harsh, but it depends what you want the outcome to be – success on the world stage, or a wider distribution and potentially less success.

Would any British athlete who has won medals on the world stage over the past twenty years say that UK Sport had been unkind to them? Of course not. They'd say we gave them every chance to be successful. In fact, I have a poster on my wall from the women's hockey team who won bronze in London, on which is written, 'Sue Campbell, thank you so much for the no-compromise approach.' Had we compromised, they wouldn't have won that medal – or gone on to win gold in Rio.

Government set UK Sport a medal target, but we needed to translate that into something that was more athlete-centred and inspirational. We talked about wanting any athlete in the UK who had the talent, ambition and work ethic to be the best in the world to be given a fair chance to succeed on the world stage. We believed that if we got that right then the medals would take care of themselves. It was no different from my approach to education: if you focus on helping young people to be the best people they can be, they'll be successful in life.

Since Katherine Grainger took over as chair in 2017 and Sally Munday replaced Liz Nicholl as chief executive in 2019, a new strategy has emerged, with money being spent on more athletes across more sports and a greater emphasis on sports having a healthy culture. The one thing I am certain of is that excellence will never be something on which you can compromise. In the recent Games in Paris

Team GB won 65 medals and finished in 7th place in the medal table.

After stepping away from UK Sport, I didn't really have a plan. I went back to the YST, but had already decided to leave there in 2017. And while I had a good working relationship with our chief executive Ali Oliver, who was and is a great professional and extremely capable, I didn't want to be under her feet. That meant I spent a lot of time out of the office, speaking to head teacher conferences and advocating for PE and school sport at the Department of Education, all over again.

I had other commitments giving talks to businesses about the Olympic performance system and how to get the most from their workforce. But I had been working for five decades, and I was well into my sixties, so I was warming to the idea of shifting into an easier life. The dogs – who are much like me, never happier than when they're traipsing through the Leicestershire countryside – would have been delighted if I had. The idea of playing more golf also appealed, as did spending more time in local village life.

Then in 2016 came a call from Football Association (FA) chief executive Martin Glenn, who invited me in to talk about the role as head of women's football. We parted without any agreement, and I flew to New Zealand a few days later with Alison Oliver. We had been invited by Sport New Zealand to take part in workshops in various cities and provide a keynote address at the Sport New Zealand coaching conference in Auckland. Martin called to offer me the job but I told him that I could not give him an answer there and then. I needed time and space to think through the thousand questions that were racing through my mind.

Did I really want another big job? Having got used to getting up, walking the dogs and maybe dropping into the YST office in Loughborough, down the road from where I lived, did I really want to be making regular treks to Wembley? Then, having decided that maybe I did want to do it, I started to question whether I had the necessary energy. When you start a new job – especially one that involves creating a whole new strategy – you need that extra-special bit of zeal, and I wasn't sure I could muster it at the age of almost seventy.

When I got back to England, I met Martin, said I'd given it some thought and was grateful to him for thinking of me, but that I wanted to start winding things down. Unfazed, Martin asked, 'OK. How many days a week do you want to do?' I paused, before telling him I'd probably be happy to work three. And that I'd want to be home-based. And that I didn't want to be on any boards or attend lots of management meetings, because I'd had enough of organisational systems and structures. As I ran through my list, Martin kept nodding. In the end I said, 'Are you just going to say yes to everything?' and Martin nodded again. This was proving difficult to wriggle out of, so eventually I stopped wriggling and agreed to take the job.

When Martin asked what sort of salary I wanted, I told him that I had only ever taken roles because they helped me to change lives through sport, so I had no salary in mind. He offered me a figure and that was pretty much that. From being semi-retired a couple of weeks earlier, I suddenly had one of the biggest and most exciting jobs in British sport.

Why did I agree to take on the role? First, because I'd loved football all my life. I remembered the little girl who regularly skipped school to play football with her mates. The game was like a third parent to me. I also remembered being told that women don't play football, and I hated the idea that girls were still being told the same, well into the twenty-first century. But I also recognised the potential football had to change the lives of millions of girls and women and positively impact wider society, if its enormous power was harnessed properly. Football has its problems, but it's our national game, far bigger than any other sport, so I thought it could begin to drive a level playing field.

Women's sport has never had the profile it deserves. It's had moments, like the London Olympics and Paralympics, when lots of British women won medals and phenomenal athletes like Jess Ennis and Ellie Simmonds became household names, but then the interest largely faded until the Rio Olympics four years later. But football is a constant presence in the nation's consciousness and reaches homes that most sports and government legislation can never reach. Equal opportunity is a vague notion to many, but if someone's daughter gets into football, and they regularly see women playing, coaching, refereeing or commentating on football on TV, it becomes more concrete, more real.

On a more personal level, the job was the first opportunity I had to combine those two driving forces of my career: sporting excellence and grassroots sports development. Up until then, those two things had been stored in separate compartments in my head, but now I had the chance to create a vision and a strategy to lock it all together. Could I create that perfect circle of excellence driving participation, participation driving talent and talent driving excellence? I always believed it was possible ... now I was about to find out.

I didn't know what I was walking into at the FA, because I didn't know where they were in terms of women's football. As long as I had the energy to change even one life through sport, I wanted to be involved, but I wasn't sure how long was left on my professional battery. So the plan I had in my head was to go in a few days a week, as had been agreed, develop a strategy for women's football, hire some good people, and leave in three years or less, when I still had the legs for rounds of golf and dog walks. But when I started looking into things, and saw how much there was to do, I didn't think, 'Oh gosh, what have I done?', I thought, 'This is amazing, the potential is absolutely enormous ...'

It very quickly became clear that not much was being invested in the women's game, which meant we were dictated to by commercial sponsors. If a sponsor wanted the FA to run a few women's football festivals, we ran a few festivals. If a sponsor wanted the England team to play somewhere, they played there. There was no strategic framework, and certainly no real vision. Martin had one, to be fair to him – he wanted women's football in England to be better, and wanted someone to lead the change. That was my job, and Martin let me get on with it while being incredibly supportive.

Every few weeks, I'd pass Martin in the corridor and he'd say to me, 'Is that strategy written?'

'Not yet!' I'd reply.

'What are you actually doing?'

'I'm listening, Martin!'

Martin was only joking, but I think there was an element of, 'What is she doing, wandering around the building and chatting every day?'

By listening to people, I was finding out how things were run and what needed changing. I did my usual trick, asking the people already working on the women's game those three killer questions – What do you do? What could you do? What's stopping you? – and I discovered that while they had incredible passion for the women's game and a shared ambition to see it achieve its potential, they had not been empowered to take the lead or use their creativity (wonderfully, five of them are still working for the FA).

I'd say to people, 'Do you want to be the best?' and they'd obviously say yes. Then I'd follow up with, 'But you haven't got a system to produce the best.' Some people seemed a bit baffled by that, just as some people had seemed a bit baffled at UK Sport when I told them we needed to change.

After six months of listening, I told Martin that the women's game wasn't ready for a strategy, as there were so many areas that needed attention, from grassroots to the élite end of the game. That being the case, we agreed to write a three-year plan focusing on three main goals — doubling participation, doubling the fanbase and making significant progress towards winning a major tournament — before producing a full strategy by 2020.

When Martin asked if I wanted a separate women's division, I said no. I didn't want the women's game to be a few people in a corner somewhere; I wanted everyone at the FA to believe they had a part to play in its future and be excited about the journey. To that end, we decided that we would place one individual in every department, someone who understood what we were trying to do for the women's game and who could enthusiastically advocate for it and cope with setbacks.

I made a clear action plan for our three goals, and Martin agreed to let me recruit a number of external people to work alongside the experienced team we had internally. Building the right team is such a central part of driving change. Being excited about the potential is one thing, but just like at UK Sport I needed good colleagues to accompany me on the journey.

While the team I inherited was good — and more than capable of becoming better — I also needed people with different experience and knowledge, and a track record of success and gritty determination. Kay Cossington coached England women's youth teams and was just back from maternity leave when I first met her, and I immediately realised that she was a talent that had not yet been given the opportunity to fly. So I looked for someone who could complement her technical expertise. We hired David Faulkner, who had overseen success in women's hockey, to work alongside her. David was part of the Great Britain men's hockey team who won a gold medal at the 1988 Olympics in Seoul. David went on to become the performance director for England hockey and GB hockey. In 2017 David joined the FA as head of women's performance to work with Kay to begin to transform the women's performance system.

Kay was appointed as head of women's player development and talent in 2017. She flourished alongside David – although not in his shadow, because she's very much her own person – and together they challenged and changed the status quo. David left after the Tokyo Olympics but Kay continued to grow and develop and was appointed the FA's first-ever women's technical director in 2022.

At the same time we appointed David we also recruited Audrey Cooper; Audrey had competed in beach volleyball in the 1996 summer Olympics in Atlanta, Georgia. She went on to become head coach and performance director at British Volleyball before moving to UK Sport. We needed someone to lead the development of coaching for the women's game and she was the perfect fit. Audrey had a massive impact, built a good team and introduced new initiatives at every level of the coaching pathway. She is now working in the professional game (for NewCo) leading the development of people across the Women's Super League (WSL) and Women's Championship.

Louise Gear, who worked with me at the YST for eighteen years, was a great team leader and an outstanding grassroots sports development manager, and she also joined the FA in November 2017. She began by leading the delivery of the work to double participation and has gone on to become head of development for the FA. The work that she and her team have done to create equal access for girls in schools and clubs has been truly remarkable. Another key appointment was Marzena Bogdanowicz, who joined us as head of marketing and commercial for women's football. Marzena had been a driving force at the British Olympic Association (BOA) and led the marketing for Team GB. Her role at the FA was to put in place the plans and campaigns to double the fanbase and attract commercial partners to work alongside the women's game. We had now assembled a team to deliver the plan and we were ready to go!

A big part of leadership is identifying things you're not good at and surrounding yourself with people who can do them better, which is what I have done wherever I've been. And very quickly, we became a strong, united team, full of courageous, resilient people willing to go the extra mile for women's football.

We published Gameplan for Growth in 2017, before getting down to rolling out our programmes and driving our profile. I knew that the quickest way to increase participation was through young girls, but also that embedding programmes in schools wouldn't generate results quickly enough for our three-year plan. We discussed the idea of a community-based programme, introducing girls aged five to ten to the fun and enjoyment of football in a safe, non-competitive environment.

The marketing team, led by Marzena, did some research into names and the Wildcats centres were born, places for girls to make friends, gain confidence and hopefully fall in love with football.

Having thought very carefully about the kind of environment we wanted to create, our Wildcats coaches, who obviously knew their football, were also trained specifically to work with young girls. We all know that boys and girls need to be coached differently, particularly at the beginning of their journey. Language that motivates boys might be a turn-off for girls, and one moment of chastisement might put a sensitive girl off sport forever. Girls respond better to praise and encouragement, particularly at the early stages of development when confidence may be low.

The Wildcats centres soon became very popular, with seventeen hundred up and running by 2020. At the same time, our schools programme (sponsored by Barclays from 2019) got under way. I've always respected that the primary objective of schools is learning (with certain caveats), and head teachers are always more interested in anything with an educational angle. We also wanted to make clear that we were not in the business of chasing other sports out of the curriculum but complementing and adding value. We took time to design our programmes so that they had wider educational value beyond football.

Our primary-school programmes, developed with Disney, focused on storytelling through football, to help with literacy. Our secondary-school programmes were about leadership, working collaboratively and competitively as part of a team, resilience, self-discipline, all things that aren't just useful on the playing field, but which also provide young people with the confidence to take on whatever challenges life throws at them.

We met our target of doubling female participation in three years, which went some way to disproving the notion that it's simply not in girls' nature to want to play football. I strongly believe that the reason fewer girls play football, and sport in general, is because of the way we treat girls and boys as they develop and the constant impact of social media. We are in danger of following traditional stereotypes rather than offer all young people an opportunity to try all sports and activities, regardless of gender.

Whether girls are less competitive than boys because of nature or nurture is irrelevant: what matters is that we provide opportunities for all girls to play and enjoy the game. That's why we decided to cater for girls through four separate but linked participation strands: football for learning (teaching important life skills through football in schools): football for fun (casual football with friends); competitive football (playing organised competitive games) and football excellence. It was about providing girls with the same opportunities and support as boys, understanding their motivations, and giving them the chance to experience football in whatever way they wanted.

The number of women and girls playing football in England reached 5.3 million in 2024 up from 1.7 million in 2017. Over the same period, there was a 54 per cent increase in affiliated women's and girls' teams.

It's going to take time for female participation in football to match that of male, but that is only to be expected when so many barriers need breaking down.

I recently watched a programme which involved presenting a firefighter, a soldier and a police officer to a group of primary-school children. The twist was that they were wearing masks, and the children assumed that all three of them were men. That's how ingrained these stereotypes and biases are. Too many girls think that certain things aren't for them, but only because they've learned that from the world they live in.

Gender equality is not about everyone being the same: it means not confining people to certain boxes based on whether they're male or female; it means letting everybody do whatever fills them with passion and excitement, not what society expects them to do. Not every girl wants to play football, but thousands will suddenly realise they love it if you just give them the chance.

We also set up 150 Just Play centres for adults and almost a hundred community clubs by 2020. Again, that was about understanding that as a governing body, the FA must strive to provide all things for all people. Some women want to have a fun kickabout before heading to the pub for a couple of drinks. They're not interested in competition, or being the best, they just want to get out of the house for a few hours on a Wednesday evening, get out of breath and share a few laughs with their friends. It might not sound like much, but it's important.

I was surprised at how little attention the FA had given to promoting élite women's football – it seemed to be happening under the radar. I knew that the élite women's game had been effectively banned by the FA between 1921 and 1971, but I thought it would have developed more of an interest in the ensuing four decades. There were key women like Hope Powell (England manager 1998–2013) who tried to drive change and did undoubtedly move things forward, but she could have done so much more with the right level of funding and support. As it was, when it came to the goal of doubling the fanbase for women's football, we desperately needed to raise the game's profile.

With Marzena and the marketing team fully focused on the women's game, we began to see an increase in press coverage and TV viewing figures. There were also innovative ideas such as announcing the 2019 World Cup squad using stars from sport and entertainment, which had a big impact on social media.

In 2018 we moved to a full-time professional league of twelve teams: the Women's Super League (WSL) and a

semi-professional second tier, the Women's Championship.
In 2019 we got our first title sponsor, Barclays, and in 2021
we sold the TV rights to Sky and the BBC. That brought in
much-needed money, some of which we were able to
distribute to the clubs. The club game was moving at an
incredible pace – now it was about winning the hearts and
minds of the many remaining cynics.

One of the biggest challenges was getting people to take
women's football seriously – not seeing it as better or worse
than men's football, but credible in its own right. Thankfully,
as the game got greater exposure, attitudes started to shift. I
suddenly had men telling me how much they loved watching the women's game. One told me that he only watched
women's football now, because it was how men's football
used to be, in the good old days.

Elite women's football certainly isn't soft – some of the
tackles are very rugged (and there is plenty of fruity language,
as the wonderful Jill Scott will attest to). But they rarely
exaggerate injuries or abuse the referees. The women's
professional game is élite, competitive sport at its very best
– high-quality, robust and fair.

I knew we could change people's views because I'd heard
it happen in real time. At a WSL Manchester derby, I was
sitting in front of two regular followers of the men's game.
Before kick-off, I overheard their conversation, which wasn't
very complimentary. 'What on earth are we doing here?' said
one, and the other replied, 'Don't worry, we'll watch the first
half and then make a polite exit.' When the officials, who

were all women, walked out, it was, 'Good grief! Are you looking at this? What a farce . . .' But when the whistle went and the teams got down to it, I could hear that their attitudes were changing.

What they appreciated, apart from the standard of football, was the lack of foul play and play-acting. Then, about ten minutes in, there was a bit of a fracas, and the referee stepped in and sorted things out, firmly and without protest from the players. One of the old boys said, 'Brilliant! We could do with her in the men's game on Saturday.' Bit by bit, perceptions were evolving, not only about women as footballers, but also about women full stop.

Men's football is a multi-billion-pound business and attracts an enormous number of fans. Naturally, there is much to learn from it, but it has many features the women's game shouldn't copy. Male footballers are distant figures nowadays. It's hard for the person on the terraces to relate to their eye-watering salaries and lavish lifestyles. In contrast, one of the great emerging strengths of the women's game is the relationship between players and fans.

The women who play at the élite level are so relatable. It's not that they take their football less seriously than the men – they want to win matches, and they certainly don't like losing (much like me!). But they are authentic and accessible, they want to be good role models for young people, and they take their responsibility for growing the game very seriously. The women's game is family-friendly, attracting new and different fans (or customers, to use modern sporting parlance), and providing often thrilling theatre for all to enjoy.

The challenge is to retain that special culture as more broadcast and commercial money rolls in. We talk about 'treasuring our treasures', understanding our history and heritage, respecting the game for all it could contribute to society, and it being a beacon of inspiration and hope for millions of girls and women. That's the stuff that will really matter as we grow.

13

Creating a platform for success

Building the right systems and employing the
right people are the keys to success

The journey towards achieving success in a major tournament was more challenging, and as much about the clubs as
it was about the England women's team.

Some clubs, such as Arsenal, Manchester City and Chelsea,
already had full-time professional players, but we needed to
raise the standard of play across the board and attract international talent. So in 2018, we decided to open the licence
again, which sets down the expectations and regulations of
operating a club at the professional level. We offered existing
clubs the first opportunity to apply and then opened it up to
other clubs after that.

All the clubs had to apply for a licence for tier one (for full-
time professional league level) or tier two (for part-time
professional league level), which wasn't universally well
received. For example, Doncaster Belles had a great history,

having won the old Premier League National Division title twice in the 1990s, but couldn't afford to pay players, which ruled them out of the running.

I had a meeting with all the clubs and was completely up front. 'If I was in the shoes of those who cannot make the journey,' I said, 'then I would be really angry with me too.' I understood their pain and disappointment, but my job was to do what was right for the whole of the women's game. I'm sure Doncaster had an effigy of me that they stuck pins in. But it came down to integrity, doing what I believed to be right, not what was popular or expedient.

I was announced as director of women's football at the start of 2018, which made me responsible for the England teams, on top of everything else.

While I knew we had the potential to win a World Cup or a European Championship, my time at UK Sport had shown me exactly what world-class success looked like, so I also knew that there was a lot of work to do to create a performance environment in which dreams could be realised. When I started my new role, I said to my FA colleagues, 'One day we will be the best in the world, but you'll have to bear with me, because it will take time to build a performance system and create a platform that enables us to be the best.'

My new appointment came in the wake of Mark Sampson's dismissal as the Lionesses' manager, which was a difficult time. The FA's decision to part company with Mark came after two investigations, and there followed a third after his departure. I had got to know Mark well and had developed a good personal relationship with him. And despite the events surrounding his dismissal, I remained respectful of the success the senior women's team had under his leadership, including a semi-final at the World Cup in 2015.

Following his abrupt departure, I stepped in to take the reins. We had a couple of friendlies coming up, so I sat down with the players and told them that we needed to appoint an interim manager until a permanent manager could be found. They all wanted Mo Marley, the Under-19s coach who had handled all of them at some point and commanded their trust and respect. After everything that had gone on the players were in a bit of a slump, but Mo stepped in without a moment's hesitation and was brilliant with them, leading them to two thumping World Cup qualifying wins.

We had 147 applications for the job of permanent manager, including from many of the biggest names in the women's game. But as the list whittled down, applicants started dropping out of the process. A couple of people managing abroad seemed like a good fit, but they didn't want to move their families to England, while the media circus around Mark's departure spooked some other potential candidates. Emma Hayes, who had won two WSL titles with Chelsea, and Nick Cushing, who had won four trophies with Manchester City, did not want the job, former Arsenal boss Laura Harvey had just joined a team in America, and John Herdman, who had led Canada's women to two Olympic bronze medals, had just taken over as manager of Canada's men.

Mo had thrown her hat in the ring in case we couldn't find anyone else. When I asked her if she really wanted the job, she replied, 'Honestly? No. But I'll do it . . .' Mo was, and is, a wonderful, authentic person and a great coach, but she had no interest in talking to the media and all the other tasks that come with a high-profile managerial role, so I had no choice but to keep looking.

One day, I happened to be talking to someone about former players who had recently earned their UEFA Pro Licence, which is the highest coaching certificate available, and were just making the transition into coaching. Frank Lampard and Steven Gerrard were on the programme, and they soon joined Derby County and Glasgow Rangers respectively. But another name that came up was former Manchester United, Everton and England player Philip Neville.

Phil's first coaching stint was as an assistant to England Under-21 manager Stuart Pearce in 2013, before he joined his old Everton boss David Moyes at Manchester United. He took charge of non-league Salford City for one game in 2015, before joining his brother Gary as a coach at Valencia. When Gary was sacked after a run of three wins in sixteen league games, Phil followed him out of the door. It wasn't the most immaculate coaching CV, but people told me he was a student of the game and very keen to get better.

So one day, I phoned Phil out of the blue and asked him if he'd ever considered coaching the England women's team. 'No, I haven't,' he replied, 'but I will think about it.' I made it clear that I wasn't on a headhunting mission and that we'd have to interview him, and sent him some reading material. He came back a few days later and said he would like to be considered.

I interviewed Phil along with the FA's technical director Dan Ashworth, our CEO Martin Glenn and the head of HR Rachel Brace, and I instantly liked him. It probably helped that I knew his twin sister Tracey, a fine netball player and a very successful coach who led England to the Commonwealth Games gold medal in 2018. He was open, warm and funny, very passionate about the game, a proud family man, and came armed with a reference from David Moyes, who said he was the best captain he had ever had. We were concerned about possible skeletons in his closet (because of the Mark Sampson situation), but he assured me there were none, so we offered him the job.

Phil's appointment was not without controversy. Some, including journalists, fans and female players, had expected us to appoint a female manager. They thought the fact that Phil had almost no experience of management and had never coached women's football was proof that the women's game still wasn't being taken seriously. It didn't help when Phil described the job in a BBC interview as 'the right development path'.

One former England women's player questioned whether Phil would be able to deal with women players. When someone dug up a couple of ill-advised sexist tweets Phil had posted quite a few years earlier, the media had a field day.

They certainly made some of his early interviews quite challenging. But the bottom line was that none of the top female managers wanted the job, the players had made it quite clear that they simply wanted the best person available, and Phil was the only person brave enough to take it on.

At Phil's first press conference, he was interviewed by the BBC's Dan Roan, who asked what made him think he could coach women. Phil replied that when he studied for his Pro Licence, he'd been trained to work with players regardless of gender. The theory being, a defender is a defender, a midfielder is a midfielder, and a striker is a striker. I was thinking, 'Hmm . . .'

A couple of months later, at the SheBelieves Cup in America, Phil asked me for a chat. And the first thing he said to me was, 'Women *are* different. They constantly ask me "why?" Every practice, they want to know why we're doing things and what difference they're going to make.' I replied, 'You're right, women are different. And this is a talented group of players who want to be fully involved in every aspect of the game and determine their own destiny.'

I knew Phil would need some support as a new coach in a women's environment, so we worked very much as a team in the early days. I'd even go into the dressing room before games and give every player a final good-luck high-five or hug, because that's not something he could do. But Phil was an emotionally intelligent man with some lovely qualities, and he quickly learned how to work with women, motivate them and fill them with confidence that they could achieve.

He brought a fresh approach and the players liked him and were excited to be working with him.

I'm sure Phil was feeling the pressure at the SheBelieves Cup, because there were a lot of people doubting his ability to produce a winning team. As it turned out, England acquitted themselves well, beating France, drawing with Germany and narrowly losing to the hosts to finish runners-up, their best-ever finish.

Having secured qualification for the World Cup, winning seven of their eight games, scoring twenty-nine goals and conceding just one, England returned to America at the start of 2019 and won the SheBelieves Cup for the first time. I think that was the first time the players really thought they had it in them to win a major tournament. And not many people were doubting Phil any more.

We went to the 2019 World Cup in France full of optimism, and after topping their group, Phil's team produced the best football I had seen them play, in the quarter-finals against Norway. When Lucy Bronze scored England's third, an absolute corker, it made my heart sing and filled me with hope.

I was sitting next to David Beckham and his family, and David high-fived me when Lucy's goal went in. Those pictures went viral, or so I'm told, and I said to him after the game, 'Apparently you've made me more famous than anything else I've ever done.' For weeks afterwards, people kept asking if I'd washed my 'David Beckham' hand!

David, who was good friends with Phil and had visited

the players in the changing room at the SheBelieves Cup to wish them luck, was very impressed by our performance against Norway, but sadly we couldn't repeat the performance in the semi-finals against the United States. They scored early on, we equalised through the prolific Ellen White, but they regained the lead twelve minutes later. In the second half, Ellen had a goal ruled out for a marginal (toenail) offside following a VAR review, before captain Steph Houghton missed a penalty. Steph had the courage to step up and I would have put my house on her scoring. As it was, she and the team were devastated. And it proved that my work at the FA was not complete.

All that promise and hope had been dashed again, which had a profound effect on Phil and the squad. When people talk about player recovery, they usually mean physical rehabilitation, but there is also a need for mental and emotional recovery. But the results that followed the World Cup reflected a team whose confidence and belief had fallen through the floor.

Defeats by the United States and Spain at the 2020 SheBelieves Cup made it seven losses in eleven games, England's worst run since 2003. Phil wasn't in danger of being sacked, and he still wanted to lead England at the Euros in 2021. However, when the tournament got pushed back a year because of the Covid pandemic, he told me he wanted to leave after the rescheduled Tokyo Olympics, the home countries having agreed that Phil would be Great

Britain's coach. So, I had no choice but to start scouring the globe for a new head coach.

It came down to a contest between two female coaches with impeccable credentials. One of these was Sarina Wiegman, whose Netherlands team had reached the World Cup final in 2019 and won the 2017 Euros, and who Kay Cossington and various experts at FIFA and UEFA believed to be one of the world's best technical and tactical coaches.

After many conversations with both candidates, we decided that Sarina was a better cultural fit for the players we had. Her interview presentation was mainly about togetherness, collaboration and building a united team. And she made clear that everyone in the team – players, coaches, support staff – needed to buy into her philosophy. Sarina also had a very direct communication style, to which we felt the players would respond well. At one point I asked her, 'Is it the performance of the team you're focused on and not winning?' – and I wished I hadn't. I swear her eyes changed colour, and she leaned into the screen and said, 'Why play if you're not going to win?' I knew then that hers would be a very honest environment in which people knew exactly where they stood.

We announced Sarina's appointment in August 2020, but she couldn't join us until after the Tokyo Olympics, because of a promise she'd made to the Dutch FA. Then in December 2020, Phil dropped the bombshell that he'd accepted the job as head coach at David Beckham's Inter Miami.

I didn't hold it against Phil – I'd been involved in élite sport for long enough to know that people sometimes must make decisions for themselves – and we still speak now. He did a good job with that group of players and reached a World Cup semi-final, and in doing so proved a lot of people wrong. That said, his sudden departure did cause me many a sleepless night because we had to come up with an interim plan on the hoof.

Luckily, we'd interviewed for an assistant coach a week before Phil's announcement and had given the job to Norway's Hegge Riise, one of the best players of all time and a highly respected coach. So following talks with the players' leadership team, Hegge agreed to fill in until Sarina could take over, while former Canada international and coach Rhian Wilkinson (now Wales women's head coach) became her assistant.

When Sarina finally arrived in September, I said to her, 'It's less than a year until the Euros, so while we expect the team to perform well, we're not expecting you to be a miracle woman.' I knew Sarina was special, and I always believed that group of players had the potential, but taking charge of a group of players you've never worked with before and turning them into a team good enough to win a major tournament in the space of nine months – especially given the amount of coaching time Sarina would have – seemed like a long shot.

Sarina brought her assistant coach Arjan Veurink with her, and it soon became obvious that they were an incredible double act on the training ground. Arjan is a highly accomplished coach in his own right and was with Sarina throughout her time as Netherlands boss, and while they had clear, distinct roles, they dovetailed and complemented each other beautifully.

I'd watch the Lionesses training and notice that Sarina spent most of her time standing with her arms folded. Arjan did all the technical and tactical instruction, while Geraint Twose, another of Sarina's assistant coaches, did the warm-ups and got amongst them if the energy seemed a bit low. Meanwhile, Sarina wouldn't say anything. She'd just watch like a hawk.

Every now and again, she wandered over to a player and had a quiet word, but she hardly ever raised her voice. If you didn't know better, you'd think she was too quiet, but most of her work had already been done. It was Sarina who had led the planning of the session and signed it all off. Out on the training field, her job was to observe how the players were performing and to give individual feedback.

Sarina also wanted to divide her support team into two distinct areas: on the field (coaches, analysts and medical team), led by her, and off the field (marketing, press, commercial and logistics), led by a senior colleague.

The FA had never appointed what was essentially a general manager, but we made the case and appointed Anja van Ginhoven, who had also worked with Sarina in the Netherlands. Anja was a terrific addition to the team, providing detailed planning and organisation, and ensuring that Sarina could focus fully on the players and team preparation.

When it came to the most important business of football matches, it soon became clear that Sarina and her team weren't in the business of quelling expectations. They won her first game in charge, a World Cup qualifier against North Macedonia in Southampton, 8-0, before a 10-0 win in Luxembourg. There followed a 4-0 win over Northern Ireland, a 10-0 win over Latvia, a more competitive 1-0 win over Austria, before a 20-0 win over Latvia again, which beat the existing England women's record by seven goals (truthfully, that wasn't a great advert for the women's game, but it was one of the reasons that UEFA revamped qualification for Euro 2025, so that teams are seeded to provide more competitive qualification games and which resulted in us having to play France, Sweden and Ireland).

Sarina's team won their first trophy in February 2022, finishing ahead of Canada, Spain and Germany, all ranked in the top ten in the world, to win the Arnold Clark Cup on home soil. And they came into the Euros in scintillating form, easily winning friendlies against Belgium (3-0), Sarina's old team the Netherlands (5-1) and Switzerland (4-0). That was when I started to suspect that I was watching something very special taking place.

There's no fluff and flowery language with Sarina. In common with most Dutch people I've met, you know exactly where you stand with her. Instead of beating around the bush, she'd tell someone they weren't in the team because they weren't playing well enough. If that sounds cruel, it wasn't. She showed how much she cared by taking the time to explain exactly why they weren't in the team and what they needed to do to improve. Some players might not have agreed with Sarina's assessment, but they were never left wondering why or feeling abandoned.

Maybe the family atmosphere that Phil had created had caused some of the players to lose sight of their search for excellence, but the clarity returned with Sarina's arrival. Her direct style of communication was good for them, because it helped them understand exactly what was expected.

But while Sarina was ruthless and totally committed to winning, like all the best coaches, she was actually a lovely person, very approachable and with a nice, easy-going manner. She expected high standards from her staff, but they knew they could relax and enjoy it. She expected her players to be 100 per cent focused in training but let them get on with things away from the pitch.

Sarina was a very important part of the puzzle, no doubt, but she would readily admit that the rest of the puzzle was already in place before her arrival.

For the previous few years, we'd been working on our strategy for girls and women's football, which was much more involved than the plan. Our plan focused on clear, tangible outcomes, but for our strategy we needed to gather every strand of the game – the different kinds of participation, talent identification, talent pathways, élite competitions, the England team, coach development, referee development

– and create a complete vision of where we wanted to take the whole game.

Part of our four-year strategy, which was led by Kay Cossington and published in late 2020, was called 'Blueprint for Success' (a technical curriculum for each age group on the England pathway). Kay had spent years studying the top nations in the world, including the United States, Germany, Spain, France and the Netherlands, and produced an in-depth analysis of what England could emulate, given our distinct culture, and what we might be able to improve on. For example, talented young English players had been leaving to play American college football for years, so could we offer an alternative that would keep them at home? Kay then worked with her technical team to create a system that would see England teams competing for major trophies on a regular basis for the foreseeable future, exactly as we had done at UK Sport.

That meant understanding what it took to win at the highest level technically and tactically; having the best facilities, the best coaches, the best support staff; and building a 'club player pathway', which would help players get an education, support players already in jobs, and hopefully persuade youngsters that we could provide great education and great coaching here in England as good as anything they could experience in American college football.

It also meant developing an England way of playing, which had never been talked about before. One of the hardest jobs of a national coach is blending players from different systems, and that's going to become harder to do in women's football as the game grows and clubs develop their own styles. But Kay thought it was possible to develop a distinct way of playing within the England set-up and roll out the syllabus at all levels, right down to the England Under-15 team. That way, when a player graduated to the first team, they would know exactly what was to be expected.

A couple of months after the strategy's publication, we started building a multi-disciplinary team specifically for women, which was hugely significant.

Before then, the women's game had accepted whoever the men's game gave them. They were good people, but many of them were experts in élite male footballers, with limited knowledge of female players. And having come from the Olympic environment, I understood that good intention was not enough – we had to be have the best people available, people who understood élite women's performance, whether it be fitness, psychology, physiotherapy, nutrition or analysis.

One of the biggest issues for women's football was that too few people acknowledged that women's bodies are different from men's. For too long the attitude had been, if it's good enough for the men, it's good enough for the women. But that did not meet my expectations, because I knew that other sports had been tailoring training, nutrition and kit specifically for women for years. So while top female footballers were still wearing boots designed for men, women's bike saddles had long been different from men's, as had women's running shoes.

We had many anterior cruciate ligament (ACL) injuries in women's football, but hardly any research had been done into the reasons why. Was it the boots? Had we given enough thought to women's anatomical differences? Were women being overworked in training? Were they not getting enough rest? Were the growing demands of the domestic and International calendar overstretching our women players? There was still a great deal to learn, not just about ACLs, but also whether women were eating properly, getting the right amount of sleep, getting the right psychological support, or doing the right kinds of training at the right times to fit in with their menstrual cycles.

It's amazing that people in football have only recently started talking about the impact of menstrual cycles on performance, because it's something that most women experience. When we started chatting to players about it, we discovered that some of them were massively affected and had no idea how to manage it.

Thankfully, we managed to get all the world-class people we wanted, which was a sign that the women's game was growing up fast. The FA was already running the Pro Game Injury Surveillance Project, which analysed incidence, burden and severity of injury and illness in English men's and women's international football. And in 2021, we joined up with Leeds Beckett University and data-tracking company Playmaker to investigate the demands of the domestic game on players.

★   ★   ★

From the first day I met them, I knew we had a set of players who desperately wanted to be winners, and it was my job to create the environment to allow that to happen. It wasn't about pampering them; it was simply about giving them the best.

Someone like Jill Scott, who had been playing for England for almost fifteen years – mostly in an environment which wasn't designed to get the best out of players – appreciated how much the system had changed for the better. But a few didn't understand what it took for me to turn some of their wishes into reality. Some thought I could make things happen with a click of my fingers. Alas, it wasn't that simple.

Players would sometimes say to me, 'How come the men travel on their own plane while we fly EasyJet?' I was hearing them – but we simply did not have the budget to pay for charter flights.

I got so much over the line through sheer persistence, to the extent that I'm sure there were times when people said, 'Just give her what she wants to shut her up!' (my colleagues would say I have a way of finding money under a rock, and if there's any spare going it's true that I will be first in line). But those issues were not for the players. Their job was to play football; my job was to help create the right environment, so that their dreams could come true.

Sometimes the players would get frustrated and ask, 'Why aren't you doing something?' Leadership is about remaining positive while bearing the responsibility and pain for being unable to fix everything. It was far more difficult than they imagined. I shared their passion and admired their push for equality, but my reality was that the women's game was not generating anything like the men's game commercially – and that limited what was possible.

14

Inspiring the nation

Winning is momentary – but what you do
with the platform can be life-changing

By the time Euro 2022 was looming on the horizon, I had known some of the players for five years or longer and felt like I had a strong connection to the group. I enjoyed being around them and watching their excitement and sharing their anticipation of what was to come. These women had fought so hard against all the odds to be here, and I just wanted them to achieve their collective dream.

Georgia Stanway attended YST leadership camps for several years, so I had known her since she was a teenager and it had been terrific seeing her develop as a player and a person. The first time we took Lauren Hemp to the SheBelieves tournament in America, her dad asked me to keep an eye on her. Lauren was only nineteen at the time, and I understood his concerns and anxiety. Both of these women have gone on with great determination and hard work to become outstanding players, and both would play a critical part in those next few weeks.

Jill Scott was the oldest in the squad and embodied every-thing that was great about the women's game. She had been a gangly little girl who wanted to play football, but had to play with the boys until the time came when she was told she couldn't play any more. For many years, she'd played football for no money, before earning a central contract from the FA in 2009, three years after making her senior England debut. Scotty wasn't really built for football but was a great athlete with unbelievable endurance, had a great work ethic and was a demon competitor. She was one of the best exam-ples I'd ever seen of someone having the courage and wilful determination to be the best they could possibly be!

I suppose I saw something of myself in Scotty, because I also worked extremely hard to be the best athlete I could be and was crazily competitive. I just hoped I was half as nice a human being as she was, because as well as being uproari-ously funny and great company – exactly the same off camera as she is on – she was wonderfully caring, which is why the public fell in love with her when she appeared on *I'm a Celebrity, Get Me Out of Here!* (which I was glued to, by the way). And despite all her achievements, she never developed an ego and or lost her sense of humour or perspective.

I invited Scotty to an event a few years ago, without telling her it was at the House of Lords. When we met in the lobby of a nearby hotel, she said to me, 'Where's this gig, then?' And I replied, 'In a little place just over Westminster Bridge ...' As we rounded Big Ben, she repeated the question and I pointed at the House of Lords and said, 'In there.' 'Oh my God,' she replied, 'am I dressed all right? If I'd known we were going there I'd have brought a different suit . . .' But once we were inside, she took it all in her stride and settled right in. Scotty cared deeply about England and the women's game and really wanted to make a difference. And since announcing her retirement from the game in August 2022 she's gone on to do many special things in life, outside football.

England's captain Leah Williamson was a different personality from Jill – less comical, more serious – but no less caring and passionate about the women's game. Leah went to the 2019 World Cup as a twenty-two-year-old but barely played, which she found tough, because she was giving it all in training.

But when Sarina took over, she immediately realised what a special talent she had in her ranks. And when Steph Houghton suffered a bad injury in the autumn of 2021, Leah was the obvious choice to replace her as captain.

Leah is a remarkable footballer and is capable of doing things that not many other women players can do. People have likened her to the great Italian defender Paolo Maldini because her ball distribution, positioning and timing are superb, and she is usually able to win the ball back without making a tackle. But more than that, Leah always shows deep concern for everyone around her and is passionate about using the team's successes to improve the lives of women and girls in wider society.

The other two players who gave me such pleasure as people and were the rock that Sarina could build on in weeks leading up to the Euros in 2022 were Millie Bright and the incredibly versatile Rachel Daly. They were great friends and a constant source of generosity, humour and kindness. I had watched them both work and work at their game and felt they were in a great place going into the competition.

With women like Leah, Georgia, Lauren, Millie, Rachel and Scotty at Sarina's disposal, I started to think that maybe – just maybe – she could pull off a miracle after all.

I met up with the team the day before England's Euros opener against Austria at Old Trafford – match day minus one – and the following morning, prior to the game, we all went for a walk along the canal to the traditional coffee shop stop where everyone's drinks had been pre-ordered. I tried to sound calm and relaxed as I chatted to the players, while inside I was as nervous as I had ever been.

At Old Trafford they opened the fan zone early, because so many families were trying to get in, and it was a joyous atmosphere. It was a family festival with lots of laughter and excitement, everyone just having fun. I walked around for an hour or so soaking it all up, feeling a sense of great pride and anticipation. Could I ever have dreamed of this? No, I couldn't: it was absolutely awesome.

When I walked into the stadium, it almost took my breath away. I've always been a Manchester United fan, so I'm very fond of Old Trafford anyway. But to see it full for the opening game of the women's Euros was something else entirely. It was just a wonderful spectacle, although there was so much smoke from the celebratory fireworks I could barely see the pitch. And I felt as nervous as if I was about to play – dry mouth, heart beating nineteen to the dozen, and just so anxious for the team as they stepped out into that tsunami of noise.

I knew Austria were a good team because they'd run us close in World Cup qualifying. But the England players were unquestionably affected by the tension and expectation in the stadium and didn't play with their usual freedom. I felt like I played every ball, and I honestly could have been physically sick with the tension.

When Beth Mead scored after sixteen minutes, I still couldn't relax. England were in control for most of the match, but every time Austria went on the attack, I thought the worst. With twelve minutes left on the clock, Austria's Barbara Dunst darted down the wing, cut in and shot, forcing Mary Earps into a fine save. Thank goodness for Mary, because 1–1 would have felt very different. As it was, England held on for the win to settle the nation's nerves.

Mercifully, the group games against Norway and Northern Ireland made for more comfortable viewing, winning as we did 8–0 and 5–0 respectively. England looked like a very cohesive unit in those games, which was no accident. Sarina was a great believer in momentum and a cohesive team performance and she stayed with the same starting XI when she could, rather than chopping and changing. She also had some game changers on the bench who would come on in the second half to create new challenges for the opposition. There was no doubt that everyone knew and understood their role – from the starting XI, the substitutes and the bench players – and all played their part brilliantly.

That said, our quarter-final against Spain in Brighton was like an unusual form of torture. My FA colleagues said it was more entertaining watching me than the game at times. Spain were excellent from the first whistle, controlling the ball and setting a frantic pace that England often struggled to keep up with. When the Spanish scored after fifty-four minutes, I thought this cannot end here – we must find a way. In Sarina we trust!

One of the things I most admire about Sarina is her calmness under pressure. She rarely stands on the touchline, and you never see her shouting at her players and the officials. She remains in the dugout, constantly reviewing the game. The only time she enters the technical area is when she wants to pass on a tactical instruction. And now, with England twenty-five minutes from being knocked out of their own tournament, she made a couple of cool but bold substitutions, replacing Ellen White and Beth Mead, who had scored seven goals between them in the group stage, with Alessia Russo and Ella Toone.

With six minutes remaining, Lauren Hemp floated a lovely cross into the box, Alessia nodded it down, and Ella Toone lashed in the equaliser. It felt like my heart was going to jump out of my chest.

Then, six minutes into extra time, Georgia Stanway received the ball in acres of space just inside the Spanish half and carried it twenty yards, before scoring a stunning long-range goal that took me from torture to bliss in a heartbeat. It wasn't just that it sealed a semi-final spot for England: it was also proof that this team had the belief as well as the skill to win the tournament.

When I saw Sarina running onto the pitch at the final whistle, roaring and shaking her fists, I really believed we could win the whole thing. And I think a lot of people in England thought the same. She knew what a big game that was, because there was no better team than Spain left in the tournament.

By now, something special was brewing across the country. The BBC had done a brilliant job covering every game and the crowds were incredible (the record for total attendance at a women's Euros, set in the Netherlands in 2017, was broken with fifteen games remaining). Our game against Spain had attracted over nine million TV viewers and streams, the team were front- and back-page news, and they were all over social media, for all the right reasons.

When I arrived in Sheffield for our semi-final against Sweden, the city was one big sprawling, happy party. A few Bramall Lane regulars told me they'd never experienced an atmosphere like it. To me, it felt a lot like walking through the Olympic Park for the first time at London 2012.

Sweden had only narrowly beaten Belgium in the last eight but were ranked second in the world, so it shouldn't have been a surprise that they were the better side for the first twenty minutes and created a couple of chances that they failed to put away. It was only once Beth Mead put us ahead that we settled, before taking complete control after the break. Of course, the goal everyone remembers is Alessia's outrageous backheel that made it 3-0. It exemplified the confidence and freedom Sarina had instilled in the players. And like Georgia's goal against Spain, it was trending on social media for days.

After the final whistle, the stewards couldn't get the fans to leave because they were so high on happiness. I am sure some of them are still there! The players' connection with the fans was incredible, an authentic joy that spread throughout the stadium, a moment for all of us to savour.

I remember watching Ellen White's tears of joy and celebrations. She had been such a key part of England's team for so long and had played a central role in our success in 2019, only to see our hopes dashed by the USA. This was a very special moment for her personally and for the team as a whole. They had made it all the way to a major final and now it was all to play for against England's great rivals, Germany.

Before the final, I had a chat with the FA's chief executive Mark Bullingham, who replaced Martin Glenn in 2020. We spoke about a friendly against the Germans in 2019, when we'd both been in the tunnel before kick-off. Mark had commented on how assured the Germans looked, which somehow made them look physically bigger than the English team, even though they weren't. Meanwhile, the English players were shuffling from foot to foot and stealing nervous glances at their opponents. Neither of us was surprised that Germany won that game.

I knew Seb Coe when he was the best middle-distance runner in the world, and he always exuded confidence (some would say arrogance). He strutted onto the track and never looked in the slightest bit flustered. As he once said, every time he went to the line, he knew he wasn't going to lose, and his rivals knew they weren't going to win. That's the kind of self-belief you need to be the best in the world at anything. And at Wembley in 2022 it was the English women who looked more assured and bigger than the Germans.

Sarina and her support staff had created something special, no doubt about that. The detailed analysis of the opposition, the sports psychologists' work with the coaches, the players' physical conditioning, the medical team's planning . . . All of it had been world-class. And they'd taken a determined, talented group of players who weren't quite sure of themselves and turned them into a united, focused team who were going to give everything to deliver in front of their adoring fans, families and friends. Like Seb, they knew that if they performed to their maximum potential, they weren't going to lose – and they'd land a major tournament win for England for the first time since 1966.

Waiting for kick-off, I couldn't help thinking back to my days playing sport for my country. Back then, I had to buy my own kit, or borrow it and hand it back after the game. Sometimes, I had to organise my own travel and find my own accommodation. And because I wasn't the best player by a long way, I warmed an awful lot of benches. But when I pulled on that shirt bearing my country's name and flag, it was an unmatchable feeling of fulfilment.

Similarly, when I heard the national anthem that evening at Wembley – 87,192 people (minus the German fans) singing 'God Save the Queen' – I got the same goosebumps and dry mouth I used to get before a netball international. I felt so connected to the moment. Alive, vibrant, immensely proud.

People ask me if I enjoyed the final. No, I didn't. It was very far from enjoyable; it was absolute agony. I don't get sweary or aggressive watching England play, but I do get very involved. One journalist described watching an England match with me as 'a tense affair', while people have learned not to sit anywhere near me, because I constantly elbow them in the ribs. In fact, various ministers have complained about the bruises they've sustained.

When Germany's top goal scorer Alex Popp withdrew after the warm-up, it surely shortened England's odds. But Germany had won the tournament eight times, while England had only beaten them twice in twenty-seven games. The only time England had reached the final before was in 2009, when Germany hammered them 6-2. On the other hand, we had beaten them 3-1 at Wembley a few months earlier, so it was possible. But I still felt horribly anxious.

It was a nervy, niggly first half, and the best chance fell to the visitors: a German player flicked on an in-swinging corner, Leah Williamson blocked Marina Hegering's effort on the line, and there was a bit of confusion before Mary Earps finally dropped on the loose ball. Cue blessed relief. England's best chance came just before the break, when Ellen White combined with Beth Mead down the right wing and Ellen lashed the ball just over the bar.

Germany started the second half stronger, with Tabea Wassmuth shooting straight at Mary when through on goal and Lina Magull flashing the ball wide after some lovely inter-play (I should say that these descriptions might not be accurate because I watched most German attacks through my fingers . . .).

Then, just after the hour mark, the incredible Keira Walsh received the ball deep in her own half and played a long, raking ball worthy of Glenn Hoddle in his pomp, right into the path of Ella Toone. Ella, who had only been on the pitch a few minutes, had a German defender coming up fast behind her, but coolly chipped the ball over the advancing goalkeeper to give England the lead. That sent Wembley into raptures. However, German teams don't tend to roll over so we knew we were still in for a fight.

First, Magull rattled a post with a ferocious shot that had Mary beaten; then, with eleven minutes remaining, the same player stole in at the near post and poked the ball home to send the game into extra time.

One of the most talked-about moments of the final was Scotty's sweary outburst having been fouled by Germany's

Sydney Lohmann. I won't repeat what Scotty said, but I'm told you can buy mugs emblazoned with her words. On a serious note, I think the public reacted so positively to her outburst because it demonstrated just how passionate and competitive these women are – how much it matters.

Anxiety turned to terror in extra time, like nothing I'd experienced before. Germany's men had broken English hearts so many times in the past that suddenly it seemed eminently possible that their women would do the same.

Then, with ten minutes to go before a dreaded penalty shoot-out, England won a corner. Lauren Hemp swung the ball into the box, Lucy Bronze nudged the ball forward off her thigh and Chloe Kelly, on as a substitute, swung a leg and missed. It looked like the chance had gone, but Chloe reacted quicker than the German defenders and poked the ball home at the second attempt. Cue pandemonium across the nation. I could have run around the Royal Box swinging my top around my head, just like Chloe was doing on the pitch.

When the final whistle went, I felt like I'd reached the top of a very tall mountain. I was shattered, but beyond ecstatic. At times, my work at the FA had felt like trying to push water up a hill. But all that effort, all that pain, all those disappointments and frustrations, became worth it in that moment.

The first person I bumped into on the pitch was Sarina. She said to me, 'What have we just done?' I hugged her hard and replied, '*You've* just won the Euros for the second time on the trot, that's what you've just done! You really are a miracle worker!'

Sitting alone on the podium, while the players did their lap of honour, I checked with myself that it wasn't a dream and tried to make sense of it all.

I was very fond of those players and wanted it so much for them. For some, it had been a struggle just to be able to play the game they loved; many of them had had their dreams shattered at previous tournaments. So to have a ringside seat and be able to witness their joy was beautiful. Those players deserved the very best – and we'd done everything we could to make sure they were surrounded by the very best.

It made me think of that time I got a terrible school report and told my dad how I'd never amount to anything in life. If you remember, he said to me, 'Sue Campbell, you will be whatever you want to be. You just haven't decided what it is yet.' That lesson has driven everything I've done since. And while I couldn't play for England at Wembley, as I'd hoped, and it was the players who had won the tournament, I'd helped make it possible for these wonderful women to achieve their dream.

Then I looked up at the fans, all smiling, singing and dancing, and thought, 'I wonder how many lives we've changed today, how many flames we've lit in children's hearts. How many girls will leave this stadium dreaming of playing for the Lionesses and believing they can be a champion one day?'

And then I thought, 'I'm really, really hungry' (I'd barely eaten for two days). On reflection, the beer I had in the changing room was a big mistake ...

15

Better never stops

*Sustained success comes from a restless
desire to go to the next level*

The post-match party ran well into the night, and I don't
remember much about it other than dancing with Sarina's
dad. As you can imagine, most of us were feeling a bit
rough on the ride to Trafalgar Square the following morning, where thousands of people were waiting to toast the
players. So when Leah Williamson and Lotte Wubben-Moy
tapped me on the shoulder my first thought was that someone was ill.

'Sue,' they said, 'we don't just want to be remembered for
winning the Euros, we want to be remembered for what we
went on and did with it.' Well, I could have burst with pride:
when they might have been singing their heads off and
enjoying a few glasses of wine, they were thinking about
their responsibility to the girls' and women's game. It was
selfless beyond belief.

Having explained that they wanted girls to have the same access to football as boys in schools across the country – because there's not much point in inspiring girls if they're not able to play the game – I suggested they write to the two prospective Prime Ministers, Liz Truss and Rishi Sunak (Boris Johnson having resigned shortly before the Lionesses won the Euros).

Once the dust had settled, Leah and Lotte drafted a letter that all twenty-three squad members signed, and off it went to Mrs Truss and Mr Sunak (although it was also posted on the Lionesses' social media channels, so that neither leadership candidate could ignore it).

Here is their stirring letter in full:

Dear Rishi Sunak and Liz Truss,

On Sunday evening history was made. The dreams of twenty-three women came true. England became European Champions for the first time in history.

Throughout the Euros, we as a team spoke about our legacy and goal to inspire a nation. Many will think that this has already been achieved, but we see this only as the beginning.

We are looking to the future. We want to create real change in this country and we are asking you, if you were to become Prime Minister on 5 September, to help us achieve that change.

We want every young girl in the nation to be able to play football at school.

Currently only 63 per cent of girls can play football in PE lessons. The reality is that we are inspiring young girls to play football, only for many to end up going to school and not being able to play.

This is something that we all experienced growing up. We were often stopped from playing. So we made our own teams, we travelled across the country and despite the odds, we just kept playing football.

Women's football has come a long way. But it still has a long way to go.

We ask you and your government to ensure that all girls have access to a minimum of two hours a week PE. Not only should we be offering football to all girls, we also need to invest in and support female PE teachers too.

Their role is crucial and we need to give them the resources to provide girls' football sessions. They are key role models from which so many young girls can flourish.

We have made incredible strides in the women's game, but this generation of school girls deserves more. They deserve to play football at lunchtime, they deserve to play football in PE lessons and they deserve to believe that they can one day play for England. We want their dreams to also come true.

This is an opportunity to make a huge difference. A change that will impact millions of young girls' lives. We – the twenty-three members of the England Senior Women's

Euro squad – ask you to make it a priority to invest in girls' football in schools, so that every girl has the choice.

Regards

The 2022 UEFA Women's EURO England Squad

After winning the Tory leadership election, Mrs Truss came to an England training camp in London. It happened to be my birthday; Georgia started a chorus of 'Happy Birthday', and the PM happily joined in. Later Leah and Lotte sat down with her and the Secretary of State for DCMS and reiterated everything they'd said in their letter. Mrs Truss reassured us that she would take it away and give it serious consideration. And off she went. Ten days later, Mrs Truss resigned, soon to be replaced by Mr Sunak. As luck would have it, Mr Sunak had already written back and had promised to address everything the team asked for, which gave us some hope.

Over the following months, I had meetings with various people, and took Leah and Lotte with me when I spoke to Education Secretary Gillian Keegan. Leah in particular spoke with incredible eloquence. When Mrs Keegan started talking about sport being good for your health, Leah said, 'Yes, but it's not just good for your health. Where do you think my leadership skills came from? My confidence? My communication skills? My ability to collaborate as part of a team?' She went through a long list of all the things that sport had given her, and I sat there thinking, 'This woman is so special.' Leah has the capability to do whatever she wants after football, and her visit to a refugee camp in Jordan in

2023, followed by a speech at a United Nations summit where she addressed gender stereotyping and argued for a level playing field for girls, provided a clue.

However, as is often the case in politics, nothing seemed to be moving very quickly. We did not want to make a public fuss, because the government already had some major issues to deal with, not least the economy. In the end, the FA's policy advisor Rebecca Besalel said to me, 'Can you manage a big round of meetings? Because if we're going to get this over the line we need to get in a room with all the influencers and decision makers.' So off I went, meeting every special advisor, chairs of the select committees, MPs, anybody she managed to get me in front of. She really did do an incredible job.

In March 2023, the government announced that it was investing £600 million in PE and school sport in a two-year period. In addition, schools would be required to offer equal access to sports – not just football, but all sports – and deliver a minimum of two hours' PE a week. When I told Leah and Lotte before the announcement was made, they were so excited and proud of what the team had achieved.

Persuading the government to take that action was a wonderful example of élite sport and élite athletes making a difference at the grassroots level, and I think I can safely say that that group of women will be remembered for a lot more than their famous victory at Wembley.

Of course, the Lionesses stand on the shoulders of so many pioneers of women's football, who spent years battling against suspicion, disinterest and outright hostility. When I was a child, women's football was effectively banned by the FA, and many women in the team that won Euro 2022, particularly the older ones, had to put up with all the same challenging prejudices.

In the past few years, the so-called Lost Lionesses, who played for England at an unofficial 1971 Women's World Cup in Mexico, have finally had their story told and been commemorated (the team of mostly teenagers, one of whom, Leah Caleb, was thirteen years old and four feet ten inches tall, played against the hosts in front of ninety thousand spectators at the Azteca Stadium – and were handed suspensions by the FA after returning home).

Meanwhile, we tracked down every woman to have played for England since 1972 and presented each one with an England cap with their own personalised number. Some of them came to talk to the current players and described the various indignities they'd experienced, including constant mockery from men, having to wear hand-me-down kit and juggle playing with paying jobs. And at the 2024 National League final at Luton Town's Kenilworth Road, women who played in the first-ever Women's European Championship final at the same ground forty years earlier (losing on penalties to Sweden) were presented to the crowd at half-time. It's so important that we value and celebrate those amazing women, because without them women's football wouldn't be where it is today.

A peak TV audience of 17.4 million people watched the Lionesses beat Germany in the final of Euro 2022, while more people watch WSL highlights than men's English Football League highlights. The Manchester derby on Sky Sports in March 2024 had a peak audience of 589,000, a record for a WSL match on pay TV (as a comparison, the opening weekend of the men's Championship, which set a Sky Sports record, had an average of 631,000 viewers across all four matches), while Chelsea vs Liverpool in November 2023 attracted the highest-ever average TV audience for a WSL game: 796,000.

In the 2023–24 season, the WSL set a new attendance record with thirty-six games to play. Arsenal's game against Manchester United in February attracted 60,160 fans, another WSL record, and the Gunners sold out the Emirates in back-to-back matches, outstanding work by their marketing team. The Lionesses regularly attract more than seventy thousand fans when they play at Wembley – 83,000 watched them beat Brazil in 2023 – and they usually sell out other stadiums, including Coventry City's Building Society Arena and Bristol City's Ashton Gate, which hold 32,000 and 27,000 people respectively.

As soon as we came out of the Euros, Mark Bullingham called me in and said he wanted me to lead on setting up the new independent club-led body to run the top two women's leagues, the WSL and the Championship. That sounded fairly simple when he said it, but it turned out to be quite a complex project.

The FA doesn't run any of the top divisions of men's football in England, and the only reason we ran the women's leagues and invested heavily in them was because nobody else wanted or had the capacity to do so. But the FA concluded that it would be better for the women's game if it stepped aside and allowed the clubs, who were co-investors, to have a much bigger say.

I started by speaking to the chief executives of every club, none of whom I knew at the time, about what they thought this new organisation, which we provisionally called NewCo, should look like. In the meantime, we began an extensive recruitment and interview process to find the new CEO. Our preferred candidate was Nikki Doucet, a former investment banker and general manager of Nike womenswear in the UK. The club chief executives felt we were travelling too quickly and that we needed to get greater clarity on the ambition and vision for the new entity before appointing the CEO.

I gave Nikki the choice either to lead a series of CEO workshops to crystallise the vision or take a step back and re-enter the CEO competition at a later stage. Much to her credit she said she wanted to lead the workshops, knowing that this could either work for her or against her! It was a courageous decision indicative of Nikki's great integrity, determination and ambition.

We invited all twenty-four CEOs to a meeting in London to discuss the way forward. I had prepared some slides but didn't get too far before it became obvious that this forum wasn't going to solve anything! We decided to establish a smaller working group, representative of both leagues, and asked for volunteers. To my delight nineteen CEOs volunteered to engage in the process and we identified ten who provided us with the mix of clubs and interests across the two leagues. Nikki then began a year-long round of workshops. She called the process 'Project Moonshot', to set out the innovative and challenging adventure on which we were all about to embark! Nikki did a brilliant job of helping the club CEOs to appreciate the distinctive nature of the women's game: same rules, different fans, different players and different needs.

We did some fan insight and found that less than 20 per cent of people who came to watch women's football went to watch men's football, which meant that 80 per cent of them were new customers. Who were they? How did we reach them? How should we communicate with them? What did they want their experience at the game to be?

Nearly all the workshops were attended by all the CEOs, and together we hammered out NewCo's vision, which is captured in the phrase 'Women's Football Transformed'. Nikki was confirmed as the NewCo CEO at the end of 2023, and it was agreed that it should take over the running of the WSL and the Championship from the FA on 1 August 2024.

The club CEOs were aware that there needed to be investment ahead of revenue and that it might take ten years of investment before NewCo started generating the kind of income that would sustain the women's game. But they remained positive and bought in to both the ambition and the vision.

Nikki's ambition is to transform the top two leagues into a commercially successful business, but the clubs will need to play their part financially. A few Championship clubs not affiliated to men's clubs could be left behind if they are unable to find investors. American businesswoman Michele Kang, who recently bought the London City Lionesses, has described NewCo as 'like a start-up tech company in Silicon Valley', meaning at this point it is about believing in the ambition and being willing to finance the incubation of the business. Other independent clubs might struggle to attract the same kind of forward-thinking investors. As harsh as it might sound, that's the price of taking women's football to the next level.

Nikki has appointed a small senior executive team and we have appointed an independent Board to run the company. But to fulfil the ambition, NewCo will also need to forge more partnerships and attract more sponsorship – easier said than done. Women's sports have traditionally attracted lower levels of sponsorship and broadcast revenues despite the growing popularity and huge growth potential. The clubs themselves will also need to increase match-day revenues, which will require more teams playing more regularly in main stadiums, more investment in marketing and constant promotion of the women's game.

As I said at my first FA board meeting, 'The men's game is like an oak tree, in that it stands out in the forest. It's tall, it's powerful and it seems like it's been there forever. The women's game is a sapling sitting beneath the oak tree, and my job is to dig that sapling up and replant it in the sunlight, so that it can grow into the tree that it really wants to be.' I could see everyone looking at each other as if to say, 'Who is this crazy woman?' But that's what we've done: dug up that sapling and replanted it in its own sunlight.

Whatever tree it becomes we want to protect the essence and culture of the women's game. It has a distinct identity on and off the field of play and it is essential that this does not get lost as the game becomes more commercially driven and high profile. We want women's football to be a welcoming place, a safe place and a happy place.

Our biggest ambition is for the WSL to become a league that every female player in the world wants to play in – but not just because of the size of the salaries. We want them to come because we create the right environment and they feel valued and that their health and well-being as players and people is central to all we do.

Our data shows that we get more families watching women's football, which makes for a very different, distinctive atmosphere. Many men's football fans support the team that their fathers and grandfathers supported before them. They belong to 'a tribe', giving them a strong sense of belonging which can be both a good and a bad thing. At best they have a loyalty to their club regardless of results and support the club through thick and thin. At worst the tribe becomes aggressive and taunts the opposition, creating quite a hostile and uncomfortable environment. Women's football also has a younger fanbase, which means it's potentially a lucrative, long-term revenue stream. Clubs will also tell you that because most people who support their women's team are new and unique, they sell more merchandise when the women play at their main stadiums.

I believe that sport reflects society, but also that society can reflect sport, especially football. That's why I want women's football to model the best of what we want to see in our youngsters, and that means players and coaches setting a good example with their values and behaviours, as well as demonstrating great skill, athleticism and competitiveness.

The women's game can learn a lot from the men's game commercially, but the on-pitch behaviour needs to reflect the unique values and behaviours of women's sport, which is distinctive from the men's game. It's important that coaches and referees are treated with respect and demonstrate great respect for one another. A big part of good leadership is about setting a good example with your values and behaviour. And we need more women leaders in all walks of life.

I've been in sport long enough to understand that the passion of the moment can make people do things they wouldn't normally do, but just because successful male coaches go crazy on the touchline doesn't make it right, however successful they are. How can it be right when it incites players, staff and fans of both teams? Sarina Wiegman and Gareth Southgate – who resigned as manager of the England men's team after the 2024 Euros – always manage to keep their emotions in check and remain dignified under extreme pressure. They have both done an outstanding job for England and brought great pride and success for the nation.

As a young person I was a terrible loser, the kind of child who would tip the board over if I was being beaten at Monopoly, but as an adult I now recognise that sport is not a matter of life and death. Losing is painful, but I believe we learn more from our failures than we do from our successes, and it doesn't make you a bad person if you lose. Women's football should portray models of behaviour we would like young people to emulate: for example, when England beat Belgium 6-1 in 2023 and the Belgian players formed a tunnel and clapped the English players off. Most people thought those days had gone, so it was a special moment: sport as it should be.

Maybe I'm being unrealistic, but if the women's game goes the same way as the men's, it will become a second-class sport, a pale imitation of men's football, instead of a proudly distinctive entity – a place that showcases what women are capable of and inspires a generation of women to become active and fulfil their dreams.

Greater professionalism will undoubtedly lead to a better product on the pitch, and the standard has already improved massively in recent years. Women's football in England had been quite rigid, with a stubborn adherence to 4-4-2, but it has become much more fluid. Watch Sarina Wiegman's England team and you'll see wing-backs coming right up the pitch, forwards switching wings, the goalkeeper spraying passes all over the pitch, all while rarely leaving holes, because midfielders know when to drop deep and protect the defence. It's quite beautiful to behold, like watching a brilliantly choreographed dance.

The better the quality, the more coverage the sport will get, and the more famous players will become. Even a few years ago, who would have thought that women footballers would win the BBC's *Sports Personality of the Year* two years in a row, as Beth Mead and Mary Earps did in 2022 and 2023? But it's so important that those players remain authentic and relatable because they will be role models for girls and women, and I know they take that responsibility seriously.

Many of the reasons for women and girls being reluctant to do physical activity are the same as when I studied the subject at university in the early 1970s. A recent This Girl Can survey found that a lot of women and girls still feel too self-conscious about their bodies to exercise in public, still equate being competitive, sweaty and muscly with masculinity, and have experienced men laughing and verbally abusing them. And now they have the internet to deal with too.

Social media has caused millions of women and girls to feel uncomfortable in their own skin (men and boys as well). They're bombarded with filtered pictures of friends and celebrities and stick-thin models and brainwashed into thinking that's what females are *supposed* to look like. But as Mary Earps recently said in an interview, 'There's more pressure than ever before to look a certain way, which portrays this unrealistic version of what society views to be attractive.'

The reality is that women and girls come in all different shapes and sizes, and the notion that there is only one way to be any woman, never mind an attractive one – is incredibly regressive.

That's where women footballers can – and do – help. Several Lionesses have spoken candidly about their struggles with body image issues and how playing and excelling at sport helps them feel more content with how they look in the mirror. As Mary Earps puts it, 'We all wish we could change some things [about our bodies], but I just try to celebrate the fact that my body can do incredible things and set an example for young girls watching me.'

That's what sport should be saying to everyone – be happy with who you are.

Having said that, there is a paradox in women's sport, in that while female athletes are generally more comfortable with their bodies, they experience specific body-focused pressures due to playing sport. Leah Williamson has spoken about how she feared missing games at Euro 2022 because of her endometriosis and the painful periods that characterise the condition, which left her curled up on the bathroom floor unable to move. And a 2022 UK study found that a significant number of players questioned displayed eating-disorder symptoms, which is a concern shared by many sports.

For a sportsperson to be the best, everything has to be perfect, which means you're going to have to think about weight and body shape. But coaches and support staff must understand that women and girls are generally more self-conscious about how they look than men and boys, and there is a big difference between educating female players about proper nutrition and so-called fat shaming. A couple of years ago, Fara Williams, England's most-capped player, said fat shaming was common when she was playing. If I ever heard a coach calling a player fat, I'd give them a piece of my mind.

Acceptance of women as athletes has come a long way, but the amount of misogynistic nastiness the England players get on social media is horrific. Has society got worse? I suspect it's more the case that social media has made it far easier to abuse people, most of the time without any consequences.

Even one negative comment can be upsetting, so what must hundreds of people commenting on someone's appearance do to that person's self-esteem? It doesn't even bear thinking about. And when the abuse is incited by individuals who should know better it is even more distressing. Irrational criticism of others because of gender is totally unacceptable in the twenty-first century.

The Lionesses travelled to the 2023 World Cup in Australia and New Zealand with a much-changed squad, not by design. Record goal scorer Ellen White and the great Jill Scott had retired after Euro 2022, while that tournament's golden boot winner Beth Mead, captain Leah Williamson and experienced midfielder Fran Kirby were all ruled out with knee injuries. Meanwhile, Millie Bright and Lucy Bronze had only just returned to action after knee surgery. Sarina had her work cut out, that much was certain.

Given the difficult circumstances, England's performances down under were every bit as commendable as their performances at Euro 2022. The Lionesses had been a highly skilled, technical team at the Euros. What we saw at the 2023 World Cup was a heightened demonstration of their character – pure grit and determination – a group of women that wasn't going to lose without one heck of a fight.

The Lionesses won their first two games, against Haiti and Denmark, by a single goal, before hammering an under-par China 6-1 to top their group. Chelsea's Lauren James announced herself to the world in that game, scoring two goals, providing three assists and winning the player of the match award.

Lauren got herself sent off in the second round against Nigeria, although England still managed to scrape through on a nerve-jangling penalty shoot-out. There followed a 2-1 comeback win against Colombia in the quarter-finals, before the Lionesses beat Australia 3-1 in front of almost 78,000 fans in Sydney. That set up a final against Spain, who had been the best team in the tournament since losing 4-0 to Japan in the group stage (even though some of their best players had been left at home, following an apparent feud with their manager Jorge Vilda).

That Spain only won the final 1–0 was down to the sheer tenacity and courage of the Lionesses. When you play Spain you always know you will see less of the ball, and this game was no exception. It was tough and every Lioness ran her heart out but just could not pull back the one-goal deficit. It was painful to see the players crumpled up in tears on the pitch after the final whistle, but I was tremendously proud of their efforts.

Sadly, Spain's mesmeric performance would be somewhat overshadowed by what happened during the medal ceremony, when Spanish Football Federation president Luis Rubiales kissed player Jennifer Hermoso on the lips without her consent. What followed was a disgrace to football and to the outmoded and outdated attitudes that still exist in sport and society.

The unfortunate incident demonstrated that while women's football is undoubtedly a juggernaut that can't be stopped, things will come along that make a dent. That's just part of the battle.

We're challenging ingrained misogyny and overt sexism, the sort of stuff that goes on in every walk of life. We're challenging people with power who feel like they have the right to do anything they want without suffering any consequences. But one of the great things about sport is that we have a public platform to say, 'No, that is not acceptable. Something needs to be done.'

There are two ways to effect change for women in society: the first is for women to do what they do brilliantly and hope to earn respect; the second is to follow the example of the suffragettes by speaking up and putting themselves in uncomfortable places. Some people have argued that the reaction to Rubiales's behaviour was overblown – the entire Spain squad made themselves unavailable for future selection, Rubiales was suspended by FIFA and a criminal complaint was made against him – but I would argue that it's about much more than an unwanted kiss. The background to that kiss is the widespread misogyny and sexual violence in many countries around the world. It is only when women like the talented and brave Spanish World Cup winners stand up against these behaviours that we have any chance of changing things for the better.

Like Leah, Lotte and the rest of the Lionesses after their Euros triumph, those Spanish women understood something very important: winning and being lauded for doing so is marvellous, but it's ephemeral. It's what you do with the platform that winning gives you that makes you a special person.

What still needs to be done? There needs to be a concerted effort to increase the diversity of players, coaches and referees. This will undoubtedly be helped by the grassroots programme in schools and clubs extending the reach of the game to all girls. Girls' football is now in 75 per cent of primary and secondary schools thanks to the great leadership and tireless work of Louise Gear and her team at the FA. When Barclays agreed to sponsor the WSL and WC they also agreed to invest in our plans to embed football for girls within schools. They have made a huge difference to the opportunities for girls to play football and more importantly to improve the health and well-being of a generation of young women. However, there is still work to do to reach all schools and in particular to look at the fourteen-to-sixteen age group where there is significant drop-off in activity. This is partly driven by schools' determination to get good examination results and additional revision at the expense of other subjects in the curriculum, but also to girls' changing aspirations at this age.

A great deal of progress has also been made with football clubs establishing girls' sections and developing a clear competition pathway.

One of the other big challenges is the need for more and better facilities if we are to accommodate the growing number of girls and women playing alongside boys and men. Football clubs that were already full of boys are now being inundated with girls wanting to play, and there are clubs that have gone from forty girls to four hundred in a relatively short space of time. But other clubs say they're unable to accommodate girls at all because of the squeeze it would put on training facilities and pitches at a weekend, or that their coaches have no experience of working with girls. It's an area that my successor will need to get hold of, and I'm confident they will.

The support and investment in the women's talent pathway still need a great deal of development. Unlike the men's game, which has academies attached to professional clubs where boys as young at eight are recruited into the talent system, we do not have the investment or desire to develop a similar system for the girls.

We have created three rungs on the talent ladder to identify, develop and nurture talented young women from every community: Discover My Talent, Emerging Talent Centres and Professional Game Academies. The aim is to increase diversity by reaching into local communities, expand the reach by reducing travel time and increasing local provision, and support girls to fulfil their potential and for those with the ambition and talent to play professional football and hopefully represent their country.

All in all, I think we've got the talent pathway right, and Kay Cossington has to take much of the credit for that. What Kay has created is effectively a conveyor belt of talent, which is crucial if the Lionesses are to stay on top. The blueprint for success created by Kay and her team has provided the framework for the development of all England age-group teams all the way through to the seniors. Sarina has been a highly successful England manager, but international managers can only stay successful if they keep being provided with quality players.

At the élite end of the game, I have no doubt that there will be many challenges. One of the biggest questions the clubs will have to wrestle with is whether to continue playing women's games in smaller four-to-five-thousand-seater venues, usually shared with non-league men's or academy teams, or switch to main stadiums in a bid to increase revenue. It is important when games are played in the main stadium that there are sufficient fans to provide a great atmosphere. Arsenal have played five games at the Emirates and attracted nearly sixty thousand fans to each game. Bristol City played all their home games in the main stadium and had an average attendance of seven thousand. Each club is growing at a different rate and the fanbase is increasing all the time. Some clubs like Brighton are planning to build a new stadium specifically for the women's team. It's hoped that having their own stadium in the heart of Brighton will increase investment and support, and it would certainly send out a powerful message to the local community that its women's football team, while distinct from the men's, is every bit as valued.

As for the international scene, the authorities need to ensure we manage the women's calendar carefully. The potential of the women's game has been recognised by FIFA and UEFA and they are looking to provide new events and competitions which means the women's calendar is getting more and more congested. Between 2021 and 2025, there will have been two Olympics, two Euros and a World Cup, plus WSL and Champions League fixtures. This has resulted in player burn-out and an increase in injuries.

The massive increase in ACL injuries is a very worrying trend – an estimated 195 élite players suffered ACLs in eighteen months between 2022 and 2024 and as many as thirty players missed the 2023 World Cup with ACLs, including, of course, England's Leah Williamson and Beth Mead.

UEFA has announced an expert panel in a bid to gain a deeper understanding of why female footballers are more susceptible to ACLs, which is welcome (a recent academic paper revealed that in sport and exercise science research, only 6 per cent of studies were done exclusively on females). However, many suspect that one of the main reasons is staring us in the face. Fifpro (the International Federation of Professional Footballers) recently reported that too many games and insufficient rest had contributed to more female injuries of all kinds. We need to understand that the women's professional game is still evolving and that the intensity of training and matches has increased massively in the last few years. Players need to be managed carefully by club and country, and we need far more research into the impact of the game on the female body.

As Sarah Walsh, former Australia international and head of women's football at Football Australia put it, 'For a long time, women have been treated like little men.' If the people running women's football don't speed up the process of treating women like women and putting them at the centre of every decision they make, they could end up damaging the players and the product. Fans want to see the best players in action, not sitting up in the stands with their leg in plaster.

I'm sometimes asked if the women's game will ever be as big as the men's game. I think it will be just as popular, but with a different group of people: girls and young women who are inspired by the authentic, relatable, talented footballers on display; families who want to enjoy a great sporting occasion together and people who simply want to belong to a sport that represents women's place in society.

If we can keep the women's game distinctive, which will be a challenge, it has an incredible future.

Besides women's football, I have been heavily involved in disability (grassroots) and para (élite) football for the last few years. My early days at the East Midlands Sports Council and my time at UK Sport working with the Paralympics had given me a working knowledge of the issues and challenges in this area. I was asked to review the culture survey that had been carried out in 2020 and realised that there was a great deal of work needed to reshape the programme and to find greater investment. After some changes in personnel, we appointed Catherine Gilby as the new head of para football in 2021. Cath had worked for a decade with British Para swimming where she was head of sports science and sports medicine. Her passion and mission for this work burns very brightly and she is leading a significant cultural change across all the seven England para teams. The biggest shift is to move the teams from great participants to high-performance players. I recall the difference between the Paralympics in Athens 2004 and the same event in London in 2012: disabled people participating in a major sporting event transforming into sportspeople with a disability competing at the highest level on the world stage. All players regardless of ability or disability have a right to dream of playing in major tournaments and achieving world-class success. Our job is to enable them to follow that dream. There is still much work to do in this area and lots of prejudice and barriers to overcome, both within and outside football. I have every faith in Cath and her team to drive the change needed.

16

The right way – and the easy way

If you want to make an impact you have to have the
courage and determination to swim upstream

Following discussions with CEO Mark Bullingham in September 2023, the FA announced that I'd be stepping down from my role in 2024, giving us plenty of time to recruit the best person to take over from me.

I think it is important to recognise that when you are an agent of change it is both emotionally and mentally draining. There is an expression that sums this up well: 'Every good warrior needs a rest.' Looking for the person to take on this leadership role proved challenging, but an appointment has been made and Sue Day (presently Chief Operations Officer RFU) will have started work in December 2024 – rather later than I had hoped! However, I am personally delighted to be handing over to someone I respect and admire, and who will bring her own brand of leadership and energy to the job.

I will be leaving behind an incredible group of colleagues (the FA now has over one hundred people working on the women's game, compared to a handful when I joined) and an exciting new strategy for 2024–28. I know that the FA will continue to make a huge impact, inspiring positive change for women and people with a disability through football. The final major piece of work that remained for me to complete before I departed was the successful launch of the new company – the Women's Professional League Limited – to manage the professional women's game. I am delighted to say that the New Company was incorporated in August 2024 ahead of the start of the 24/25 season. A land-mark moment for women's football in England and a new exciting chapter for the development of women's football across the world.

So, what are my reflections on my incredible journey through sport? I have to begin by paying tribute to my parents. You don't realise how great parents are until they're no longer there and you're much older and wiser. And one of my great sadnesses is that I never really told them how much they meant to me. I think they knew I loved them, because I was very tactile, but there was so much I wanted to say to them after they were gone, when it was too late.

From Mum I got humour and lightness, and the ability to see the best in people and situations (not that I've always managed that). She never gave in to the dark side of life, which was what was so wonderful about her. Dad was more reflective, could see dark as well as light, and he had so much wisdom. I've still got a picture on my wall of the three of us with Charlie the dog, when I was six or seven, and I'm looking at Dad with so much love. He was a good man and very special to me.

When I was on *Desert Island Discs*, I dedicated the song 'Music Of My Heart' to my parents. Mum and Dad allowed me to be the person I wanted to be, and they crammed my heart full of beautiful music: a love of people, a love of the outdoors, a love of sport, all those things that have kept me sane and happy throughout my life. Because I grew up in such a wonderful family, it feels strange not to have had my own. Sometimes, especially now I'm older, I see people with partners, children and grandchildren and feel a pang of regret. Someone I loved dearly once told me I was married to my job, and they were probably right. I put all my energy and emotions into my work, and didn't have anything left with which to sustain a close personal relationship.

But if I could live my life again, I don't think I'd do anything different. The most amazing opportunities came my way and I tried to make the most of them. And while work was all-consuming, it was unbelievably rewarding.

On reflection, I have managed to create a feeling of 'family' wherever I've worked. We all want to belong, and seek out places where we feel like we belong, even if it's just the local pub. And I've been incredibly lucky that in every job I've had, I've been surrounded by great people who also became great friends. When I was with the Lionesses, I felt like I was part of a family on an incredible journey together. It fed that need in me to nurture, in a way I'm sure parents feel about their children. It gave me the emotional sustenance I needed – and it allowed me to belong to a special family of wonderful people.

When it comes to leadership, I've always seen myself as more of a coach than a manager, be that coaching people or coaching systems. Management is a science – setting work programmes, managing budgets, appraisals, business planning, strategies – but coaching is about people, more of an art form. And I learned coaching from some of the very best in the business: Sheila and Ron Bassett when I was at school; Eileen Alexander at Bedford; Bob White at Leicester; Rod, Rex and the rest of the team at Loughborough; all those visionaries I worked with at the National Coaching Foundation, who knew how to draw out the very best in people.

I like to think I am an invitational leader: someone who invites you to be part of achieving a compelling vision. Instead of assuming people will follow you, I share the development of the vision and the mission, so that everyone involved has a sense of ownership. I make clear that it's *our* vision and mission, and show what could happen if we all take the journey together, shoulder to shoulder. Everyone in an organisation, whatever their role, needs to feel valued and respected and play their part.

Too many people think that their lives are inevitable and unchangeable. But I believe in free will, and that we are all capable of ploughing our own furrow, our own path, through the world.

From conversations I've had with athletes, I know that – regardless of the influence of their coaches – greatness sits inside them. It's not something that anybody else can gift them. At the same time, how often they train, how hard they train, how intelligently they train, is down to them. And I sincerely believe that it's possible to help most people understand that if they make the right decisions, they can find that greatness and change themselves for the better. It's essential to facilitate that as a leader of systems: if your people don't know what greatness feels like, how can they help create an environment that will find and nurture greatness in others? Everyone can make a difference in their own world and in their own way: they simply have to decide what difference they want to make.

To get the very best from people – to draw out that greatness – you have to build relationships. And to build relationships, you must genuinely love people and show that you care. I think those girls at Whalley Range High School saw that I cared. And everywhere I worked after that, I've 'walked the job', meaning I'd spend lots of time talking to people, getting to understand them and care about their life outside work. People have lives beyond what they're doing in the business and that can affect their productivity and effectiveness.

Making time for people is central to quality leadership. Some people might say that they've got more important things to do, but caring about your troops is the most important part of a leader's job. At the FA, I was known as the 'chief hugger' – Phil Neville would say, 'There's nothing like a Campbell hug!' It has become clear to me over the years that people may forget what you said or even what you did, but they never forget how you made them feel.

I also do plenty of homework before meeting new people. If you assume that you're going to have instant chemistry with someone and don't do any preparation, you're going to end up in some awkward situations. It's the same with speeches. Because I don't use notes, it looks like I'm talking off the cuff. People sometimes say to me, 'Wow, no notes. Did you even prepare?' I smile and think of what Eileen Alexander would have said: 'You can only look like that if you've prepared really well.'

Enabling people to be the best they can be is about developing an environment in which they can learn from you but express themselves in their own way, using their own creativity; it's about collaboration and letting people work things out for themselves, but always being there when things don't go as planned. 'Roots to grow and wings to fly!'

Like the time the Lionesses wanted to write that letter to Rishi Sunak and Liz Truss: I didn't say, 'Tell you what, I'll draft it for you and you just put your names at the bottom.' They drafted it themselves. When they were happy with it, we sent it. And it was the players who were at Downing Street to take the accolades. That's what real leadership looks like: your troops out there in front, you making their lives as rich as they can be.

Seeing people grow has been one of the great joys of my life, whether it's young people from inner cities, athletes or colleagues for whom I've tried to create fertile environments in which they can thrive. I've seen so many people who have had the courage and willingness to learn and strive to become a better version of themselves. That is never an easy journey, but I'm so proud of the people they have become and what they have achieved. We often feel that we don't have control of our own destiny, but I believe we determine our own fate and that the manner in which we conduct ourselves in good times and bad is what defines us.

I've often wondered, 'How on earth did I end up here?' I've never really been able to fathom that out, except to say there has been a lot of serendipity involved and I've never strayed from my mission. There's nothing special about me – but from childhood I had a desire and a passion, which was sport. And if everyone used their desire and passion to try to improve the lives of others, the world would be a better place.

At the end of my days, I'll certainly want to know that I did my best to improve the lives of those around me. I've never had a strong religious belief, but I do have a strong moral purpose. That makes me determined and resilient and means I won't take no for an answer. I'm a paradox, because on the one hand I can't stand disharmony – if my mum and dad had a falling out, which was rare, I'd run between the rooms trying to sort things out and make the world happy again – but on the other hand I've created a lot of dishar-mony by being a disruptor.

People tend not to like change; they prefer to keep doing what they're doing because it makes them feel comfortable and secure. But if you want different outcomes, you've got to change how things are done. When I was CEO of the National Coaching Foundation, I disrupted the entire coaching education system in England and met with resist-ance. But that resistance slowly turned into acceptance, which slowly turned into application. At the Youth Sport Trust we created a new PE and school sport system across the country that challenged the status quo.

When I joined UK Sport, people thought that finishing tenth in the medal table was fine, but we needed to do better than that and we started dismantling and rebuilding the high-performance system. Martin Glenn asked me to join the FA precisely because he knew I'd disrupt things. He didn't know how, or if it would be successful, but he was prepared to back somebody who was going to tip the system on its head. We should never be afraid of challenging the past and embracing new ideas and new ways of working. Without that we stagnate!

When you're an agent of change, you can be a bit of an irritant. And I was a bit of an irritant. Some colleagues have called me a fiery presence, and I'm sure I was chal-lenging to work with at times. I'm never satisfied with the pace of change, even if things are happening at a decent speed. And there are times as a leader when you have to be steely-eyed and come across as formidable, while never forgetting that one of the most important parts of leadership is fairness.

You have to accept that in creating the change you think is right, you're not always going to be popular. And for the most part my approach has worked. Give me a big challenge and I'll work at it and work at it and usually deliver. I might struggle to tell you how I managed to deliver: it just comes from a genuine belief that I can. Having a clear mission, constancy of purpose and an indomitable will to succeed can move mountains.

Chances rarely come on a plate – you've usually got to fight for them. That's why I often say to people, 'Don't ever look back and say, "I wish I had gone for that" or "I wish I had tried harder."' I hope those who worked alongside me felt empowered, and understood that while I could be challenging, it was only because I was trying so hard and cared so deeply. It was never about me: it was about trying to change the world through sport.

Who would have thought that a mischievous little ginger-haired girl could have had the life I've had? I've met the most amazing people, from all walks of life; I've travelled the globe; I've had a ringside seat for some of the greatest moments in sporting history. And I've never lost sight of the fact that not everyone is as privileged and as lucky as me, which is why I've never stopped reaching out and trying to give people hope. I truly believe in the power of optimism, a belief that the impossible can be made possible, that challenges will be overcome and you can realise the vision.

I hope that people appreciate that everything I've done has been out of a passionate belief in my mission. I haven't always been perfect, but I gave the very best in every job I had. Hopefully I've created a legacy for sport – women's sport in particular – that will last long after I've gone. Sport has been great to me, and I hope I have served it well . . . And will continue to do so!

Acknowledgements

How lucky I was to have a loving mum and dad who gave me the music of my heart: a love of people, a love of the outdoors and a love of sport. They were two very special people.

My sister Gillian is different to me in so many ways but she too was trailblazer in her own right. Thank you, Gill, for always being there for me in good times and bad.

Sheila Bassett, my physical education teacher at secondary school, who signposted me towards becoming a physical education teacher. Without her I would never have knuckled down at school and who knows how my life would have panned out.

Eileen Alexander, the grand dame of Bedford College of Physical Education, was a remarkable woman and a great role model. Eileen had to be formidable to succeed and showed me what was possible.

Although they never knew it, and probably never will, the girls from Whalley Range High School cemented my mission. They showed me that sport could change lives for the better empowering young people to do well in life.

The University of Leicester's Bob White was my first real mentor as an adult, and he didn't just make me a better teacher and coach, he also made me a better human being.

Lecturing at Loughborough University gave me a brilliant foundation for the rest of my professional life. It helped me be a far better teacher and transformed my coaching style. A massive thank you to Rod Thorpe and the entire African violet team – a very special time.

Peter Warburton from the Sports Council East Midlands region persuaded me to pound a tougher beat in the inner cities for four years. Always there with wise counsel and great advice.

Jean Vorderman was a great friend and wonderful colleague during my ten years at the National Coaching Foundation. Of the many people I met during my time at the NCF, Frank Dick, Geoff Gleeson and Rainer Martens warrant special mentions as each gave me a special insight into great coaching. Thanks to Katie Donovan for the inspiration and leadership of Champion Coaching that showed the power of national leadership and local delivery.

Without Sir John Beckwith, there would have been no YST. His investment and commitment gave us the opportunity to grow in to a powerful movement for change in school sport.

Steve Grainger worked alongside me at the NCF and the Youth Sport Trust, we made a great team and much of what we achieved at the YST was down to Steve's unmatched sport development expertise.

There's not a lot of love for politicians nowadays, but during my time at the YST and UK Sport, I was incredibly lucky to work with some fine conviction MPs who genuinely wanted to make the world a better place. Tony Blair, Estelle Morris, Tessa Jowell, Richard Caborn, Andy Burnham and Jeremy Hunt all played their part in supporting me to drive systemic change.

The team at UKS — Peter Keen, Liz Nicholl, Tim Hollingsworth and John Steele — bound together by one mission were brilliant colleagues whose dedication and skill made everything possible.

At the FA, another amazing team of colleagues whose passion and determination drove us through some tough barriers. Thanks to all, particularly to my two CEOs, Martin Glenn, who took a chance on a grey-haired Baroness to lead women's football and to Mark Bullingham for all his support for the 'naughtiest' member of his senior management team.

To my dogs — Ben, Willow, Bronte and Kelsey — whose unquestioning love and loyalty have kept me sane in times of stress and madness.

Finally, thanks to everyone involved in creating this book, including the brilliant Ben Dirs, my wonderful agent Ruth Cairns, as well as Andreas Campomar, Holly Blood, Beth Wright, Aimee Kitson, Chevonne Elbourne, John Fairweather and the rest of the team at Little, Brown.